Primary Health Education

Beverley Young

*British Council, Nigeria, Indonesia and London
and UNICEF, Kathmandu, Nepal*

Susan Durston

*Overseas Education Unit,
University of Leeds, England*

Longman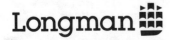

Longman Group UK Limited,
Longman House, Burnt Mill, Harlow,
Essex CM20 2JE, England
and Associated Companies throughout the world

First published 1987
Second impression 1988

ISBN 0 582 77924 3

Set in Linotron 10/12pt Plantin

Produced by Longman Group (FE) Ltd
Printed in Hong Kong

Acknowledgements

More than a decade ago, when working for the British Council on a Primary Education Project in the north of Nigeria, my colleague and friend, Hugh Hawes, pointed out that there was an urgent need for a book about health education for primary teachers. We never managed to write it but, some years later, Nigel Speight (a paediatrician working in Tanzania) and I tried to put the idea into practice. However, the time was not ripe; health education was still very much on the periphery of the curriculum.

Still more years went by and I became involved with the CHILD-to-child programme at the Institute of Child Health in London. David Morley who was the inspiration behind this brought together doctors and educators in a powerful alliance which must be one of the most significant developments in health education. I am conscious that I have learnt far more from him and CHILD-to-child than I have contributed and many of the ideas in these pages are derived from that programme.

Indeed, anyone who writes a book like this must be acutely conscious of how little original thinking it contains. I have to thank many people, some of whom I mention by name below. But there are many more unnamed, particularly in those countries where I have lived and worked for long periods of time (Kenya, Nigeria, Indonesia and Nepal), by whom I have been influenced or whose ideas I have consciously or unconsciously adopted.

In particular, I must thank:

- My friends from the CHILD-to-child programme, David Morley, Hugh Hawes, Duncan Guthrie, John Webb, June Carlile, Juliet Gayton, Paula Edwards, Mary Johnston, Marie-Therese Feuerstein and Rhylva Offer for their wisdom, friendship and imagination; also David Werner (of *Where There is no Doctor*) who participated in several CHILD-to-child meetings and whose originality, dedication, humour and skill were a constant source of inspiration
- Gill Knight, Humphrey Munga, Hamisi Mboga and several primary teachers in Mombasa, Kenya, who enabled me to try out many ideas from this book in primary classrooms
- Jackie Menczer and Joseph Toluhi who made many helpful comments on the manuscript, especially on format and organisation
- Felix King who read the manuscript so carefully and made detailed comments both on technical content and language use
- My UNICEF colleagues in Nepal, especially Carol West and Audrey Aarons, who have commented on the text and contributed to my understanding of health education problems
- Rex Meyer and the New South Wales Department of Education's Health Education programme for their concept of health as expressed in the diagram in the preface to this book
- My friends at Longman, especially Rob Francis, for their strong support, advice and patience in waiting for this manuscript
- My wife and family for their encouragement and comments, especially my son, Tim, for helping to invent the origami oral rehydration cup in Chapter 5

- My wife for preparing the Index
- David Morley for writing the Foreword
- Finally, Sue Durston, who half-way through my struggles with this book, agreed to be a co-author, producing first drafts of many of the chapters and always rendering wise comment and advice on the rest of the text. Without her, I am quite sure that it would not have been completed.

Beverley Young Kathmandu, Nepal 1986

Publishers acknowledgements
The Publishers are grateful to the following for permission to reproduce photographs:

Camera Press for figs 2.19a and 4.1b; J Allan Cash for figs 4.1a and 10.11; John and Penny Hubley for figs A2, 3.3 and 3.4; Picturepoint for figs A3, 2.19b and 4.4; John Reginald for figs 2.12; Teaching Aids at Low Cost for fig A1; UNESCO for fig 3.14; WHO for fig A5.

All remaining photographs not acknowledged were provided by the author.

The Publishers would like to acknowledge the Appropriate Health Resources and Technologies Action Group (AHRTAG) for their permission to use illustrations based on the drawings of Don Caston and Joan Thompson.

The Publishers and Teaching Aids at Low Cost (TALC) are grateful to the Swedish International Development Authority for assistance in the production of this book.

We would also like to thank the Institute of Child Health for their kind permission to use their CHILD-to-Child material.

CHILD-to-Child readers.
Also dealing with the CHILD-to-Child theme are the CHILD-to-Child Primary Health Readers. This series has been developed to teach and encourage primary school children in Africa to become concerned with the health and development of their pre-school brothers are sisters.

The books have been graded into two reading levels and each deals with a different health topic.

Titles in the series:

Level 1	*Level 2*
Good Food	Down with Fever
Accidents	Teaching Thomas
Dirty Water	A Simple Cure

Contents

Foreword

By David Morley, Professor of Tropical Child Health, University of London, Institute of Child Health.

'Health For All By 2000.' This was the resolution of the World Health Assembly in 1978. Success in achieving this goal will depend on many sectors other than health. High amongst these is the education (particularly of girls) provided through primary schools across the world. Equally, success in education demands that children should arrive at school having escaped long periods of malnutrition, and severe disease (such as measles) which can be prevented by health workers. Health and education, I am convinced, must become more inter-related.

I know that very many teachers and their pupils will benefit from this book. I would hope that they, too, will have an opportunity to work more closely with those in health, agriculture and community development. As a result I hope that they will also experience the same great benefits that Beverley Young and I experienced in working more closely together.

Dr Young's book will be deeply appreciated by all school teachers and teacher trainers in the developing world. His dynamic approach comes through in his writing, and I am sure that he will inspire many teachers with the enthusiasm to make health education a subject that the children will always look forward to and enjoy.

Those of us who are involved in finding out the reasons for a fall in mortality in many countries, have identified literacy in the mother as being a priority.

As well as providing literacy amongst the future mothers and fathers in a community, we have also come to realise the enormous part that school teachers play in many communities in the developing world.

The United Nations Childrens' fund has identified four important measures which can now be introduced in any community even in a period of recession. These will have a significant effect in reducing the mortality of children. These issues are remembered by the acronym GOBI-FFF. These (in order of importance) stand for oral rehydration, immunisation, breast feeding and growth charts; while the three F's stand for female literacy, family planning and food supplements for small children and pregnant mothers. (See top diagram, opposite.)

The new emphasis in developing health care requires community involvement. In many communities the school teacher is a leading personality. Through this book school teachers will be able to play an even greater part in the health care of their community. I had the good fortune to work with the authors of this book on the CHILD-to-child programme so well described here. Through this programme, which started in 1979, we have learnt the importance of breaking down barriers and working more closely with other disciplines as suggested above.

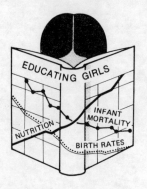

THE EDUCATION OF GIRLS IS CLOSELY ASSOCIATED WITH A FALLING INFANT MORTALITY AND BIRTH RATE AND IMPROVED NUTRITION

Priority Health Measures in Third World Countries (GOBI-FF)

1 child in 10 dies of dehydration

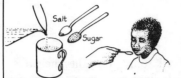

Oral rehydration for the 10 attacks of diarrhoea each child gets

Measles, Whooping Cough, Tetanus, Polio, Diphtheria and Tuberculosis

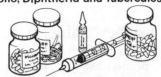

They kill five million children. Immunization prevents them all

Breast feeding and birth spacing

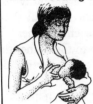

Breast feeding is important for at least two years

More births are prevented by breast feeding than contraceptives

Growth charts and good food

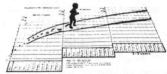

A satisfactory growth curve is the indicator of good health and nutrition

Appropriate agriculture   Appropriate education   Appropriate community development for village   Appropriate health for village

We are still in separate boxes

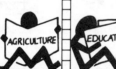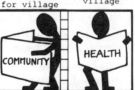

Where do we go from here?

BREAK DOWN THE WALLS

GET TO KNOW EACH OTHER

WORK TOGETHER

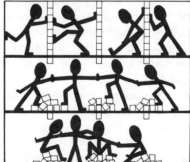

Preface

(especially for teacher trainers)

This book is for primary school teachers, especially for use in pre-service and in-service teacher training courses. However, we hope that it will also be a useful reference text for practising teachers and for curriculum planners. There is an increasing awareness among educators everywhere (both in the 'developing' and 'developed' countries) that special attention should be given to health education. Many countries now make special efforts to ensure that it has a place in the curriculum, either within science, physical education or in its own right.

Many readers of this book will not speak English as their first, or even second, language. We have therefore tried to keep the language as simple as possible. Even if training courses are in English, it is probable that another language is used in the primary classroom. At the end of the book is a glossary; it may be a good idea to teach students how to use both this and the index.

Unfortunately there is no one word in English for 'he' and 'she'. We particularly want this book to reach women teachers and to make sure that girls in primary school receive at least as much attention as the boys. We have therefore tried to choose examples which refer to girls and to use both pronouns where possible.

What is 'health'? Gandhi, that great health educator, defined it as 'body-ease', the opposite of disease. He considered health as a positive state of the body (and mind), not merely the absence of physical disease or sickness of the mind. We will use this positive interpretation of the word in this book. Especially in poor countries of the world where health problems are severe, it is too easy to

dwell only on the negative – on disease, malnutrition, drug abuse or injury from accidents.

When you think of health, you probably think first of the health of the individual person. That, of course, is important. But the term health can also apply to the environment in which people live. It can apply to the home, the school and the community. We can show this idea by a diagram:

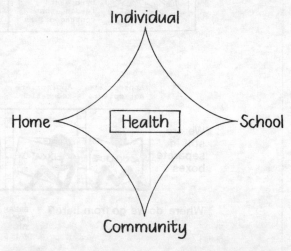

Just as you may think of the health of an individual person when you think of health, you may also think first of physical health. It is easy to forget mental health, stability within the mind ('mind-ease'), allowing a person to be at ease within herself or himself and to cope with the changing world in which we live. Many people consider spirituality as an important or even essential ingredient in this concept of mental health.

Then there is the social dimension of health. Human beings are social animals; we all interact with other human beings. Our physical and mental health is dependent, to at least some extent, on the kind of relationships which we have with others. The health of the environment in which we live is partly dependent on the actions, attitudes and beliefs of others. The ability of the human race to control and live with its aggressive instincts is perhaps the ultimate test of the social health of the planet which we inhabit. Again, we can show these three aspects of health in a simple diagram, below:

This diagram gives us a useful framework for thinking about health. In this book, you will find ideas about physical, mental and social health in relation to the individual, the home, the school and the community.

Finally, there is one most important idea which we would like to stress. In many places in the world, research has demonstrated that health education programmes which are restricted to the classrooms of primary schools only, have little impact on the general level of health of the community. Teachers have to look beyond the school – to health workers, parents, community leaders and the social services. It is only when such links are forged and the health messages learnt by children in school are reinforced in the wider community that real improvements in people's health can be expected.

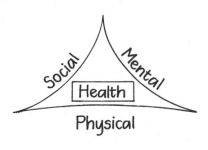

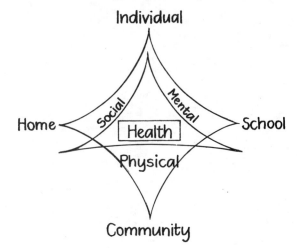

These two diagrams can now be put together:

Introduction

About this book

As you read these words, people are suffering and dying from disease, hunger and accidents. Many of these people are children. Many of them are growing up maimed or stunted in body and mind. Yet much of this death, disease and suffering could be prevented. **The knowledge exists**. The challenge to teachers is to spread this knowledge.

This is the challenge for health education.

This book is about health education. By health education, we mean education about:

- personal health and hygiene
- mental and emotional health
- community health

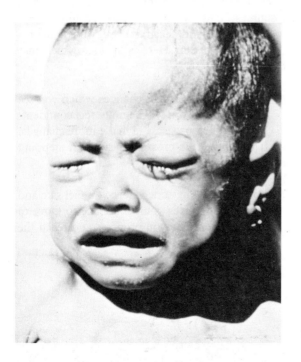 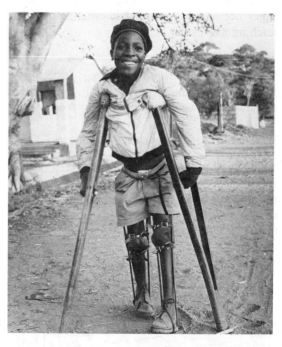

The children shown here are suffering from blindness due to lack of vitamin A (left) and polio (right). Neither of these need happen.

Through the pages which follow, we hope to share with you some knowledge, techniques and ideas about health education. Consider, for example, some of the health problems common in many countries. In this book, we shall explain:

- how a simple drink from water, sugar and salt can save the life of a person with diarrhoea
- how dark green vegetables contain vitamin A and prevent certain kinds of blindness
- how immunisation can prevent polio
- how older children can help to prevent accidents to younger children
- about the harmful effects of smoking
- how to look after teeth
- about the nutritional value of food

This is a book for primary school teachers. More especially, it is a book for those who are training to be teachers. Thus, you will find in its pages not only background knowledge but also teaching ideas such as:

- how to tell stories
- how to make lessons interesting
- how to do demonstrations
- how to use simple plays

We teach as we were taught

Think back to your time at school. What do you remember? Can you see in your mind's eye the classroom? Can you see the school and its surroundings? Which teachers do you remember? Can you remember how they taught? Can you remember what they taught you? Which events stand out in your memory? Do you remember the other children? Discuss your memories amongst yourselves and with your tutor. How do your memories compare with schools as you know them now?

A problem for teachers is that we have all been to school! The experience of school happens early in life. It leaves a big impression on all of us. From our school days we carry around with us an idea of what school should be like. In most other jobs, people come to them with fresh ideas. The power of the past is not so strong. For teachers, it is more difficult. We change slowly if we change at all.

This book suggests many ideas. Some may be appropriate for your situation, some may not. You may agree with some ideas but not with others. Some ideas may be too difficult to use because of practical problems (class size, lack of resources, cultural or religious customs). But don't give up and teach as you were taught – decide to do better! Here is an idea which may help you:

- When you make small changes which you see are successful, you will begin to feel confident. You can then progress to make more changes. It is a little like crossing a river on stepping stones.

You step on one stone where you feel safe and secure. That gives you confidence to move to the next stone. So you progress and reach the other side of the river.

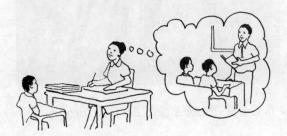

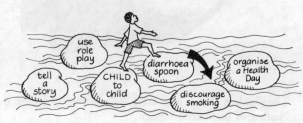

It can be like this in your teaching. You can learn to make small changes both in **what** you teach and in **how** you teach. This approach is most important in health education where new ideas may challenge deeply held beliefs. Adults, especially, find it difficult to change their ideas. They need **time** to learn and understand before they put new ideas into practice. Remember also that change needs effort. It is often easier to continue doing things as you have always done them than to change.

So remember!

make small changes
and you will cross
the river successfully

run too fast . . .
and you will
fall in the river

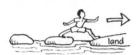
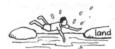

Teaching and learning about health

In the past, health education has often concentrated on changing people's behaviour. Perhaps it is more important to build upon existing knowledge and existing practice. Here are some suggestions:

- Recognise and respect what is of value already. Take time to understand and appreciate people's problems and how they cope with them. Remember that by the time children come to school they have already learnt many ideas at home. As teachers, we have to build on these ideas. For example:

- We sometimes assume that the main health problem is ignorance. We think that people do not know about good health practices. However, more often the problem is about **conflicting ideas**. That is to say, the current view of what is good health practice is different from a traditional view. The problem is not made easier by the changes in health education itself. Just as people learn a new message, the message itself changes. For example, our knowledge about diet and nutrition changes all the time. Certain diseases have become resistant to drugs. New problems arise such as the increase in bottle feeding of babies. Another problem is that 'school knowledge' may conflict with 'home knowledge'. Children can be very skilled at keeping 'school knowledge' for school and 'home knowledge' for home. Try to bring this conflict of ideas into the open. For example, encourage children to talk about the beliefs and practices of their parents. If possible, explain how these are helpful and valuable. Encourage parents to come to the school, perhaps for a special health education day (see page 199). Aim for a caring and trusting partnership between home and school.

- Needs are different in different places and at different times. For example, malaria is a serious problem on the coast of East Africa but not in the highland region inland. Mothers feed babies from bottles more often in towns then in rural areas. Certain diseases are much more common at particular times of the year. It is important, therefore, to adapt

Not
This is what you
should eat!

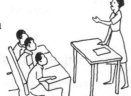

But
Let's think about what you eat at home. What did you eat yesterday? What is good about it? What is bad about it? Do you need to make your diet healthier? Why? How?

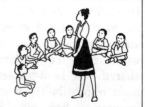

the content of your health education curriculum to your particular situation. Discuss the local problems with other teachers, the head-teacher of the school and health workers. Decide what are the main health problems. Make sure that these are stressed in the school's health education curriculum.

- Because of the way we were taught at school, we often assume that teaching means 'telling'. So teachers spend most of their time talking at children. But talking is only one way of teaching and often it is not a very good way. Try to find other methods. Because some of the ideas of health education may conflict with existing knowledge and practice, indirect methods may help. For example, stories about other people allow you to give advice subtly. Health incidents which happen to children at home or school bring a sense of urgency and reality to lessons. We often need to remind ourselves that learning is more important than teaching. We may be called teachers, but our job is to help children to **learn**.

Cooperation is the key

Teaching can be a lonely job! Of course, as a teacher, you are – or will be – with children. But how often do you see other teachers teaching? How often do other teachers visit your classroom? How often does the head-teacher visit your classroom? Even if they do visit, do you benefit from the visits and, if so, how?

Walls between classrooms are necessary. But, too often, the walls can be barriers. They can prevent teachers from learning from each other. In a subject like health education, teachers need to share ideas and knowledge. Planning, preparation of teaching materials and the scheme of work, even the teaching of children can be **shared**. The head-teacher of the school has the main responsibility for encouraging cooperation between teachers (see chapter 10).

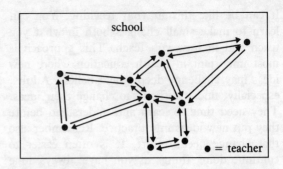

Cooperation within the school is important. But if health education is to be successful, it has to reach **beyond** the school. It has to reach outwards to:

- parents
- community leaders
- health workers
- young children who have not yet come to school
- children who may never go to school
- people who can give advice

In many countries, the primary school is the most widely distributed official institution. It has a great responsibility. It must look outwards to the community which it serves.

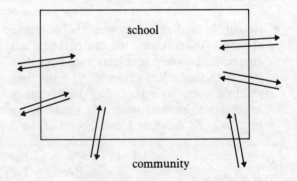

Health education in school

Consider the curriculum of the primary school. Most people will probably agree that language and mathematics are the most important subjects. There is usually less time for subjects like science, social studies and health. Indeed health education may not even be on the timetable. Perhaps it is done in science. Perhaps it is a part of physical education. Perhaps it is occasionally done during school assembly. Perhaps it receives no attention at all.

Yet we shall see in this book that the knowledge and skills of health education can save lives, prevent illness and suffering, and improve people's lives. **It is vitally important**. The authors of this book think it is more likely to receive the attention it deserves if it is a separate subject. But it does not have to be a separate subject. It could be part of the science curriculum or of 'general studies'. The really important point is that it should be **planned** and that there should be a school policy. Of course, the school policy has to be related to a national or regional policy (see chapter 10).

One important point is the effect of examinations. The exam at the end of primary school may determine a child's whole life chances. Exams have a powerful effect on what is taught and learnt in school. In most countries, there is no separate exam for health education at the end of the primary school. However, questions on health may come into the science exam or other exams. Good examination questions can help in the teaching of health. They can stress important ideas and encourage children to think. This, in turn, influences the teaching of health in the schools. It affects both the content (what?) and the methods (how?) of health education. Bad examination questions, however, are worse than no exam at all.

Find out about the exam at the end of primary school. Are there any health education questions in the science paper? If so, what are they like? Are they multiple choice or short answer? What content do the questions cover? Do the questions encourage children to think? If so, how?

Using this book

This book is in two parts. **Part I** (chapters 1 to 7) covers the knowledge, skills and attitudes of health education. Each chapter gives background information and then provides some teaching suggestions. We have not usually indicated the level at which these suggestions may be appropriate. Occasionally, however, we say that they are 'for younger (or older) children'. Particularly during a teacher training course, it is useful to consider how you might use, develop and extend these ideas. Pages dealing with Teaching Suggestions have been flagged by a grey strip down the edge of the page.

Part II (chapters 8 to 11) is mainly about methods of teaching the ideas and practices of health education and about health education in and beyond the school. Chapter 8 suggests general methods such as how to use stories, songs, drama, games and teaching aids. Chapter 9 is called CHILD-to-child. It explains how you can encourage older children to look after the health of younger brothers and sisters and other younger children. There are many occasions in health education where the CHILD-to-child idea may be used. We use this symbol in the text to draw attention to it:

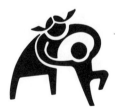

For further explanation of this powerful idea turn to chapter 9. Chapter 10 is concerned with the organisation of health education in the school, how to plan a scheme of work, how to make the school a healthy place, and how to help sick children. Chapter 11 gives some practical suggestions about how the school can reach towards the community.

A final word

We hope that you will find this book useful. However, we hope even more that you will add many more ideas of your own. For this book is just a beginning or a starting point. It is a collection of ideas, techniques, and thoughts about health education. We hope that you can use some of the suggestions as they are, and that you will adapt some and extend others. Challenge what we say. Discuss the contents of the book with other students if you are in training, or with other teachers if you are already teaching. Take the ideas and make them work for **you in your situation.**

Part 1
Health ideas and how to teach them

The chapters in Part 1 are divided into sections. The section 'Useful Background Knowledge' is addressed to you as a teacher (or student who will be a teacher).

The section 'Some Teaching Suggestions' contains ideas for use with children in primary schools. These pages are marked with a light grey strip in the margin.

Chapter One

Ourselves

Useful Background Knowledge

How do we see ourselves?

To be healthy, you need to know yourself. You need to understand your **physical** body. You need to understand your **mind**. We need to ask these questions:

- How do people grow?
- What changes take place in our bodies as we grow?
- Why are human beings all alike, and yet all different?
- How are babies born?
- Why do we feel the way we do about ourselves, our parents, people of the opposite sex?
- What makes us happy, sad or angry?
- How do we look after ourselves?

Children, especially young children, see themselves as the centre of their own world. It is difficult for them to put themselves in the position of other people. They see the world from their own point of view.

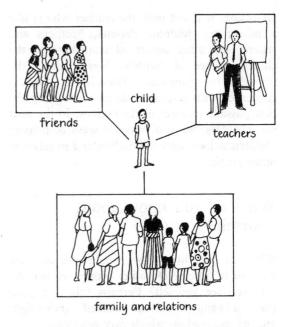

friends

child

teachers

family and relations

As a teacher you can help children to be less self-centred. You can help them to build up their own picture of themselves. You can be a little like a mirror to children. Children see themselves reflected in you. If they see that you think they are dull and lazy, this helps to make them dull and lazy. If they see that you think they are bright and hard-working, this helps to make them bright and hard-working:

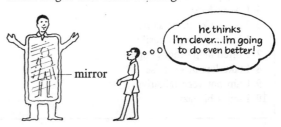

mirror

he thinks I'm clever...I'm going to do even better!

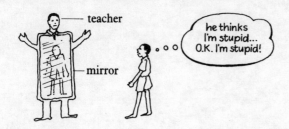

teacher

mirror

he thinks I'm stupid... O.K. I'm stupid!

Of course, it is not only the teacher who is like a mirror to children. Parents, brothers and sisters, and other adults all contribute to the child's picture of himself. Nevertheless, the teacher is very important. This chapter, then, is concerned with helping children to build up the best possible pictures of themselves. In the next two chapters, we will consider ways of helping children to look after themselves and to relate to other people.

What do you know about yourself?

What are **you** like? How would you describe yourself to others? Do other people see you the way you see yourself? Perhaps this is a good place to begin – to look at **yourself**. Above right are two suggestions which may help you:

A picture of me

At the bottom of this page is a list of statements in a table. Opposite each statement, you can show whether you agree or disagree with it. If you feel neutral about the statement, tick the middle column. **Better still, you can make up your own list of statements.**

Can you work out a way of producing a total 'score' for yourself? What does the score mean? Do you have a good 'picture' of yourself? Do any questions act as a check on other questions? If you feel you can, ask a friend to complete the same table about you! Does he or she give you the same ratings as you give yourself? How are they different? Do you think that your friend has been unfair?

Finding a twin

(This activity is particularly suitable for students on teaching training courses.)
Imagine a situation in which you discover a person who is your identical twin. He looks exactly like you. The twin lives in a different part of the country (perhaps in a town). His situation is completely different from yours (perhaps you live in a rural area where your parents are

Statement	1 Strongly Disagree	2 Disagree	3 Neutral	4 Agree	5 Strongly Agree
1 I am usually smart and well dressed					
2 I have a good figure (female) or I am well built (male)					
3 I enjoy working with other people					
4 I work hard					
5 I often like to be alone					
6 I lose my temper easily					
7 I often help other people					
8 I take lots of exercise					
9 I am not very talkative					
10 I am a bit lazy					

farmers). You and your twin like each other immediately. You talk about your backgrounds. Each thinks that the other's house sounds very exciting. You decide to change places for a few days. You also decide not to tell your families what you are going to do. However, you realise that this exchange would be impossible unless you each knew more about the other. So you decide to make a file. This file contains all the information about you which will help your twin to behave like you. Decide, perhaps with your tutor*, what this file might contain.
Below are some ideas:

What does this file tell you about yourself? Note that no other student's file will be exactly like yours. You are **you**. You are a unique person. You have your own body, qualities, talents, feelings, likes and dislikes.

To be a good teacher, you need to develop your best qualities and talents to become a mature and healthy person. Remember that your example to children is more important than what you say. So knowing yourself is very important. If you know yourself well, you can help children to know and understand themselves.

• Name	Do you have any special or 'nick' names? What are the reasons for them?
• Other people in the family	How many brothers and sisters do you have? What are their names and ages?
• Clothes	What kind of clothes do you usually wear?
• Food	What food do you normally eat? Is the food different where your twin comes from?
• Sports	What are your favourite sports and hobbies? How good are you at them?
• Jobs at home	What jobs do you do? Do your parents expect you to help at home?
• Ambition	What would you like to become? What would you most like to own? Which place in the world would you most like to visit?
• People	Who do you like and why? Which famous people do you admire most? What kind of people do you dislike most?
• Work in school/ college	What subject do you like most? What do you dislike most? Which are you best at?
• Habits	Which are your best and worst ones?
• Feelings	What makes you afraid? What makes you angry? What makes you laugh? What makes you sad?

* Footnote: *This file contains **personal** information about students. It should be regarded as their property and for their purposes only.*

Some Teaching Suggestions

The rest of this chapter is concerned with how you, as a teacher, can help children towards this understanding. It is for you to decide where in the primary school you use these ideas. Some are obviously for younger children, some are obviously for older. It would be a useful exercise to consider, with other student teachers and with your tutor, at what level you would use them.

What are our bodies like?

Ask a child to lie down on a big sheet of newspaper on the floor. Stick two or more pieces together if necessary. Draw around his body with a felt-tip pen. Get the children to label the various parts of the body.

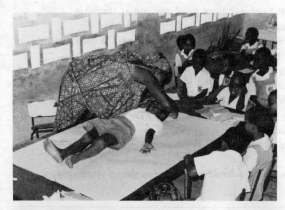

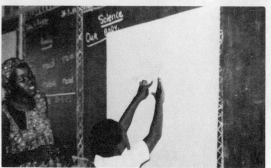

Talk with children about their bodies. You could ask them questions like these:

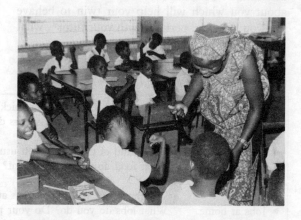

- How do you move your body? (Ask them to look at the inside of their arms and then to move their hands and fingers. Ask them what they see moving beneath the skin. The answer is a **tendon**.)

- What happens to your chest when you breathe deeply?
- Can you feel your heart beating? How many places in your body can you feel your heart beating? (The wrist, chest and neck are the easiest places to feel heart or pulse beat.)

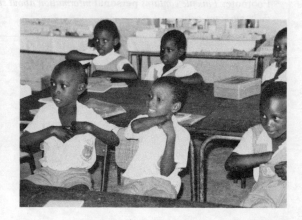

- What does your stomach feel like when it is full? Or empty?
- Can you move your eyes, your ears, your nose, your toes?
- How far can you turn round from your waist while sitting down?
- How many joints can you find in your body?
- What is your footprint like?
- What is the smallest thing that you can pick up with your toes?

There is much opportunity for good science teaching, especially with older children, as an extension of this work. You can help children to develop important skills like observing, classifying, measuring and counting.

- Let children measure around their waists and wrists with string.
- Let them count their pulse and breathing rates before and after exercise. They could record their results in the form of a bar chart or table.
- Let them classify their footprints.

How do we know about the world around us?

Talk with children about their **senses:** what they are and what they tell us. You could ask questions such as:

- What do your eyes tell you?
- Do your eyes always tell you the truth?

You could show the children a simple visual illusion like this:

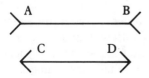

Ask the children questions like:

- Which looks longer: AB or CD?

(In fact they are both the same length. To check, the children could measure them.) Another illusion you could show them is this one:

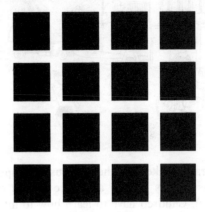

Between the black squares are white crosses. Ask the children:

- What can you see in the middle of the white crosses?

(Most people see grey spots in the middle of the crosses. This is an optical illusion. These spots do not actually exist.)

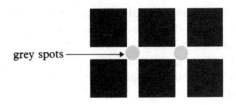

grey spots

Ask the children to look at a picture like the one shown below.

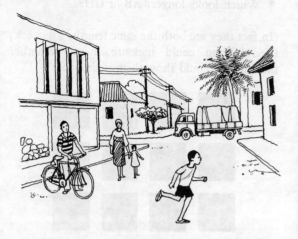

In a drawing like this, the artist uses **perspective** (that is, things further away are always drawn smaller). Children have to learn how to interpret drawings and photographs. You could use pictures from magazines and newspapers to help them to do this. You could ask the children:

- Is the child really bigger than the lorry?
- Who is nearest to the palm tree? How can you tell?

What is it like to be blind or deaf?

Let the children blindfold each other and try to walk around the classroom. (See page 54.)
   Ask the children:
- What are the problems for a blind person?
- Why do blind people sometimes beg?
- What do your ears tell you?

Take the children on a 'listening walk' and record all the sounds that you hear.
   Ask the children:
- What is it like to be deaf?
- Why are people often deaf **and** dumb?

What does your skin tell you?

Make up a 'feeling bag'. Take a bag of thin cloth or paper and put different objects inside. The children could play the game in groups. Each child makes a guess about what is in the bag. Try to find objects with different textures such as sandpaper, newspaper, exercise book paper, cardboard or plastic.

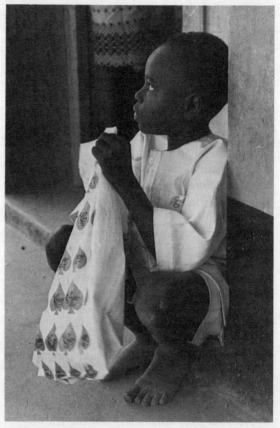

What does your nose tell you?

Make up 'smelling' boxes or tins. For details of this see page 29. With older children, get them to put in order a series of lemon (or lime) solutions of different dilutions. (For reasons of safety, it is not a good idea to encourage young children to taste unknown things.)

14

How do we feel inside?

You could draw on the board simple drawings like these:

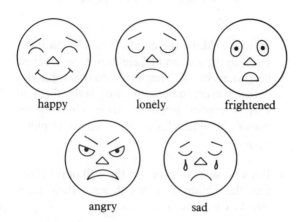

happy   lonely   frightened

angry   sad

Can the children say what emotion each face shows? (Happy, lonely, frightened, angry, sad.) They could use simply drawings like these when writing about or illustrating an experience. Let them talk with you about their feelings. Perhaps you could start by asking about:

- the clothes they like
- the people they like
- the games they like
- the food they like
- the stories they like
- the songs they like
- the dances they like
- the places they like

Remember the maths and language work which can be developed from an activity like this. For instance, find out what games are the most popular. Could this information be displayed in the form of a bar chart? What songs are most often mentioned? Do older (or younger) classes have the same likes and dislikes? What words do the children use to describe the things which they like?

Use drama where possible. You could suggest an idea to the children and let them mime how people might behave. For example, a new baby is born in the family: how do they react? How do their parents and relatives react? Groups of children could suggest situations to another group who have to act it out. Help children to realise that their feelings may not be unique. Other people feel sad, happy, angry and frightened just like they do. (See 'Ourselves and others' chapter 4.)

Growing up

From a child's point of view, growing up is a slow process. The time from one birthday to the next, or from one major event to the next, seems very long. An event like a religious festival, which is eagerly expected, approaches so slowly. It is sometimes difficult to realise (both for children and adults!) that we are changing all the time.

When we think of growth, we first think of **physical** growth. We think of ourselves getting taller and bigger. Maybe, also, we think of changes which take place as we grow. But do we remember that growing up involves **intellectual, emotional** and **social** changes? For example, as we grow the following changes occur:

- We can do more difficult school work (intellectual growth)
- We learn to control our anger, how to behave towards people of the opposite sex, and how to cope with pain and disappointment (emotional growth)
- We learn about our **social** role. We learn that we have a part to play in family life. Maybe we help our parents at home or look after younger brothers and sisters (social growth).

In many developing countries, the social role of children is very important. You could discuss with other teachers (or student teachers) and with your tutor the social roles played by children in your society. Do the roles change as children get older? How do they change? In what ways are children expected to help at home or at school or in their local communities?

Are we really growing?

We have already mentioned how, to a child, time sometimes seems to stand still. How can we help children to appreciate that they really are growing and changing? Here are some suggestions:

- Let children keep a note or scrapbook on 'Growing up'. In it, they could keep a note of how their height changes, what happens to their teeth, the size of their shoes, how their likes and dislikes change, how their faces change, and any other changes in their appearance.
- Make a growth chart and pin it on the wall of the classroom.

You can make this easily by cutting strips of paper about 4 cm wide and sticking them together. Using a ruler, mark off 1 cm

up to 150 cm
(approximately)

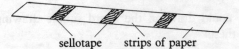

the sellotape is needed on both sides of the paper

sellotape   strips of paper

divisions. Make the chart about 150 cm high. Fix it to the wall and let children measure their heights against it. They could do this regularly, perhaps every month or two. Help them to keep a proper record in their 'Growing up books'. In older classes, children could plot a graph.

- Put a bit sheet of paper on the wall of the class. Get the children to stand with their arms outstretched and draw arcs.

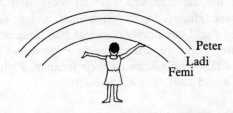

Peter
Ladi
Femi

They must all stand in the same place for the arcs to run parallel. It is important that you reassure the smaller children. Remember that they may be worried about their size. Help them to understand that they are **growing**.

- Draw some circles in chalk on the classroom floor. Ask the children to try to curl up in the middle in the smallest possible ball.

You could make it into a game where the smallest 'ball' scores the most points. Does the tallest child make the largest ball? Does the shortest make the smallest?

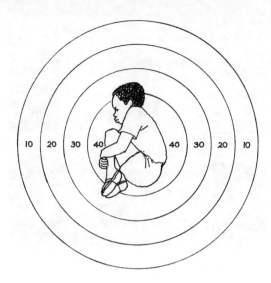

- They could measure lengths by matchsticks. Perhaps they can measure the length of their forearm or foot. Why should the matchsticks all be the same length?
- They could measure the difference between their standing height and their jump height (both with arms outstretched).

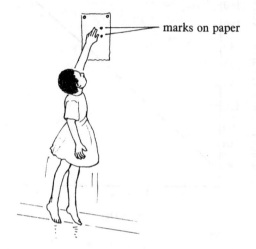

marks on paper

- Fix up two posts outside, with a bar across:

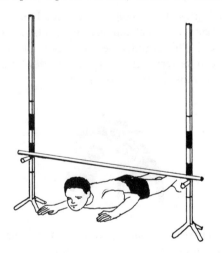

Who can get under without touching the bar? Is the shortest child also the thinnest?

The topic of growing is an excellent opportunity to do **measuring** activities:

- The children could use parts of the body as measuring instruments. How long is the desk in hand spans? Why do different children obtain different results?

Such activities can be made more interesting if children make the same measurements on their own family members. For example, you could ask them to compare their own hands with those of their father or brother and sister. They could compare:

- fingerprints (how would they take these?)
- outlines
- surface area with older children (how would they do this?)
- length of finger
- thickness of nail
- the number of seeds that could be held in one hand

Older children (in class 5 or 6 for example) could compare themselves with younger children (in class 1 or 2). They could find the average height of their own class. How would they do this? Then they could find the average height of the lower class. Cooperation with other teachers would obviously be necessary but similar data could be collected from other classes. For example, an average height graph (or bar chart) could be made:

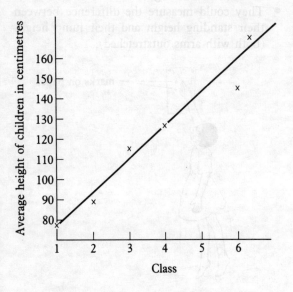

Get them to do similar graphs for boys only and for girls only.

- Are there any bathroom scales in the school? Or can you borrow one? With these, children can weigh themselves. The children could make similar weight measurements on children in other classes.
- Do any of the children have photos of themselves as babies or as toddlers and young children? You could make a chart like the one shown in the photograph.

Put the chart on the wall of the classroom. You can use it to discuss the ways in which the child has changed. Ask questions such as:

- In what ways is Caroline now similar to Caroline as a baby?
- In what ways is she different?

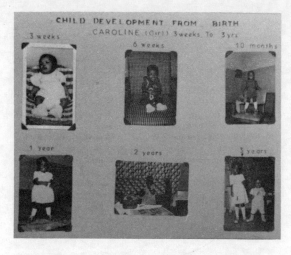

Our Babies Growing

Babies grow and change very fast. They therefore make an ideal subject for study by older children! This activity describes how older children can observe and help in the development of their younger brothers and sisters.

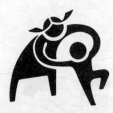

Find two long straight pieces of wood or bamboo about 130 cm long. Knock 12 nails, about 10 cm apart, into each, as shown at the top of the next page.

Number the nails from 1 to 12 on the top row and 13 to 24 on the bottom. These numbers are for the 24 months in the baby's first two years of life. The two pieces of wood can now be hung or nailed on the wall about 18 cm apart. (You could make a similar holder out of cloth if you preferred.) Now make 24 cards out of cardboard or stiff paper, approximately 6 cm × 12 cm. If

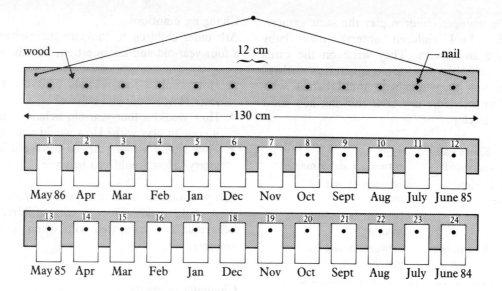

you are starting this activity, write on the first card the month one year ago. For example, if the present month is May 1985, start with June 1984. Then write on the remaining cards all the months up to May 1986. Punch a hole in the top of the cards and hang them on the nails. The completed apparatus is shown above.

Now the children bring to school news of baby brothers and sisters who were born during the past year. They write down on the card:

- the name of the baby
- the date he/she was born
- where the baby lives
- the name of the child who will be observing the baby.

The card might look like the one shown here. Use one card for each baby. You can put more than one card on each nail. In the example given, this card would be placed on nail number 12. Record children born during other months on other cards. At the beginning of each month, move every card forward to the next nail. In the example, the June 1985 card would go on to nail 13, and all the others would move up one nail.

Put a new card for June 1986 on nail 1. Now all the babies are one month older. The age of the baby in months is shown above the nail.

Ask older children to watch younger children both at home and at school. How do younger children behave? What do they (the older children) like to do which younger children don't

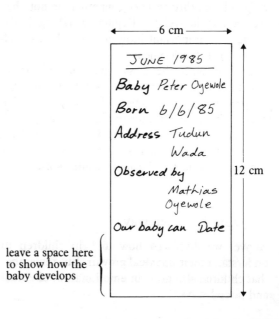

leave a space here to show how the baby develops

do? Do younger children play the same games?

The school children observe their baby brothers and sisters. They write on the cards when the babies can do certain things such as sitting up. They compare 'their' babies with other babies. Here is a table showing how most babies develop:

Most babies can:	
sit unsupported:	between 5 and 9 months
walk 10 steps unsupported:	between 11 and 19 months
say 3–4 words:	between 10 and 21 months
say a short phrase:	between 18 and 36 months

The children could write on the card other important events in the baby's life, such as sicknesses and immunisations. Check that the babies are being weighed regularly at a health or 'under-fives' clinic. Is their weight increasing? Careful monitoring of the growth of babies and young children is most important. They should be weighed monthly to check whether or not they are gaining in weight. Regular weighing is the single most important indicator of a child's healthy normal development.

Discuss with the class what 'games' babies play. Do the older children talk to them? (See chapter 9 on CHILD-to-child.) It is important that babies should be stimulated and not ignored. If you can, keep a watch on the development of the babies. If any are much slower than suggested in the above table tell the local health worker.

Growing in other ways

Above, we discussed how to help children to understand their **physical** growth. But remember that children also grow in **emotional**, **intellectual** and **social** ways.

Changing emotions

Ask older children to compare themselves with a four-year-old and ask questions like these:

- How would a four-year-old behave if he was lost? How would you behave?
- How would a four-year-old behave if he had no one to play with? How would you behave?
- How would a four-year-old behave if he was angry? How would you behave?

Can you suggest other comparisons which children could make? Discuss with children their behaviour now compared with when they were younger.

Changing interests

Ask older children to think about their interests now. Are they different from when they were much younger? (They may have to ask their parents about this!) For example, you could ask questions related to skills, hobbies, games etc.

• Skills:	Have you become better at doing things? Riding a bicycle or making a fire? Have you learnt any new skills?
• Hobbies:	Have you begun any new ones? Joined a scout troop? Have you kept up any old ones?
• Games:	Have you learnt any new ones? Volley ball or badminton?
• Choices:	Do you have more freedom to do what you want or go where you want? Can you make more decisions for yourself?
• The opposite sex	Have you become more interested in friends of the opposite sex?

More responsibilities

As children grow up, they learn to do more and more jobs for themselves and for others. As teachers, you can help children to appreciate this 'social growing'. Children could think about the ways in which they now look after themselves. Below are a series of questions which you might ask the children. Perhaps they might make drawings based on these questions.

- Can you wash yourself?
- Can you brush your teeth?
- Can you wash your clothes?
- Do you look after your hair?
- Can you get to school safely and do you always leave enough time?
- Can you cross roads by yourself?
- Do you look after your own school books?
- How do you compare in these jobs with a three or four-year-old?

They could also think about ways in which they help other people. You could ask questions such as:

- Do you help your parents on the farm or garden?
- Do you help your mother in the house and in what ways?
- Do you help at school and in what ways?
- Do you look after younger brothers and sisters at home? (See chapter 9.)

In conclusion

Remember that the ideas and suggestions in this chapter are merely **suggestions**. It is for you as a teacher (or student teacher) to decide how you can best use them with children in primary school. In which class (or grade level) are they appropriate? How can they be developed and modified for your situation? Will you use them in health education lessons, in science or during physical education lessons? They are a starting point on which you can build.

Chapter Two

Looking after ourselves

Useful Background Knowledge

In this chapter, we will consider how children can:

- look after their bodies
- look after their teeth
- lead healthy lives

Remember two important points:

The teacher's example is important
Children copy what adults **do**. If we want children to be clean and tidy, we must set them a good example. Children will not believe a person who does not behave in the way he tells other people to behave. As a teacher, your example is especially important (see chapter 11). You have to try to set a good example.

As a teacher you must be realistic
Some of the practices which we suggest here may be difficult for your pupils. For example:

- Some children come from very poor homes. Perhaps their parents are unemployed and living in the town. Perhaps their parents are farmers who have had a bad harvest. Perhaps there are many children in the family. Often parents find it very hard to afford the school uniform.
- Many children do not have piped water in their homes, or even in their villages. Perhaps people collect water from a river, or from a well. They may have to carry it a long way. People may wash their clothes in a river.
- Commercially produced soap may be too expensive for many families.
- Few children possess toothbrushes. Even fewer can afford toothpaste regularly.
- Toilets (of any kind) are still a luxury in many parts of the world.
- Many children have to walk a long way to and from school.

As a teacher you have to be aware of these problems. You have to try to understand the problems which they face. You can then adjust your teaching accordingly.

Caring for our bodies

The skin

An enlarged section through the skin is shown on page 23.

The **epidermis** is the thin outer layer about 0.1 mm thick. The surface of the epidermis consists of dead cells. They are rubbed away continuously by clothes and washing. As this happens, new cells move out from the living layer to replace them.

The **dermis** is much thicker and is made up of a network of tough fibres. Between these run blood vessels and nerves. The nerves are

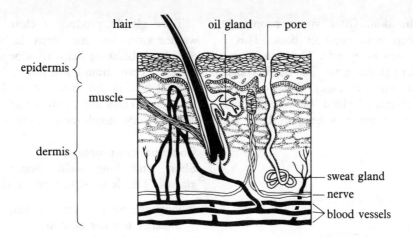

connected to tiny sense organs which 'feel' touch, pain, warmth and cold.

Hairs are a special part of the epidermis. They grow from the base of hair follicles. They cover the whole body except for the palms of the hands and the soles of the feet. Each scalp hair grows slowly for about 3–6 years. Then it rests for a few months and drops out as a new hair grows in its place. The waxy secretion of the sebaceous gland (sebum) oils the hairs and keeps the skin supple.

Nails are formed from skin-like cells also. They grow out from the nail base and gradually become hard and dead.

Skin colour comes from a pigment of the skin called melanin. It is produced by cells called melanocytes. These cells live near the base of the epidermis. They make small granules of melanin which pass into nearby cells, giving them colour. The amount and size of the granules determines the darkness of the skin.

Functions of the skin

Temperature control: The skin helps to keep the body temperature constant at 37°C. When the weather is cold, the body hair stands upright. Tiny blood vessels near the surface of the skin become narrower. Less blood flows through them, so that the body loses less heat by radi-ation. When the weather is warm or the body becomes warm from exercise, the opposite happens. The blood vessels become wider so that more blood can reach to just below the surface of the skin. So more heat can be lost from the blood. Also the sweat glands pour out sweat when the body is warm. The water in the sweat evaporates and cools the body. In genital areas and in the armpits, special glands produce a stronger smelling liquid.

Protection: The skin protects the body. It keeps out dirt and germs. If germs do enter, tiny white cells in the blood kill them. The dead cells and germs form yellow pus. Sometimes you can see this pus in a boil which eventually breaks open through the skin.

Other functions: The skin is a sense organ (to touch, heat, cold, pain). It is an excretory organ (of sweat), and it produces vitamin D in sunlight (see page 71). It keeps body fluids in. If you burn the skin, you lose a lot of fluid.

Changes at adolescence

At puberty, several changes take place in the body which affect the skin. New hormones (chemical messengers) are produced by special glands in the body including sex organs. These cause hair to grow on the body, and, in boys, the growth of a beard. New glands which produce oil grow in the skin. Often young people get pimples on their face, chest or back. This is because of the new oil glands. The skin surface becomes oily and germs grow. The dead layer of skin does not rub off easily. The openings (pores) of sweat and oil glands become blocked. Sometimes pimples can become quite large and sore.

The eye

A section through the eye looks like this:

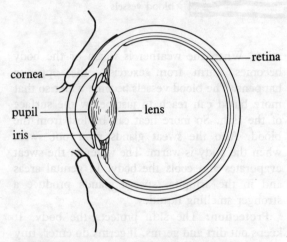

The **pupil**, the black centre of the eye, is a hole with a muscle called the **iris** around it. The iris opens and closes the pupil to control the amount of light which enters the eye.

The **lens** and **cornea** focus or point the light. As light comes through the clear cornea, it is bent a little. The lens which is behind the pupil focuses light onto the retina at the back of the eye.

The **retina** consists of nerve cells which are sensitive to light. When light strikes the retina, it makes nerve impulses go to the brain. The brain interprets the pattern of nerve impulses so that we can 'see'.

The **conjunctiva** is a thin, wet membrane (or skin) which covers the white part of the eye and the inside of the eyelids.

Tear glands produce a clear liquid which washes away dust and keeps the surface of the eye clean. Blinking helps to wipe the tears over the eye. Tears drain down into the nose through a small hole in the corner of the lower lid near the nose. Tears are produced all the time but when we cry, much more liquid is produced.

Common eye problems
Short and long sight: Some people need glasses. This is because they are either:

- long-sighted: they can see things clearly in the distance but not near to
- *or* short-sighted: they can see things clearly close to themselves, but not in the distance

Short or long sight is caused by the shape of the eyeball or lens, which makes it difficult for the lens to focus accurately on the retina. If you wear glasses, the lens of the glasses helps the lens in your eye. Thus you can see more clearly. As a teacher, you may notice children who cannot see well. Perhaps they cannot read the blackboard from the back of the class. Help them to have their eyes tested (see page 187).

'**Pink eye**' (**conjunctivitis**) is a disease where the conjunctiva which cover the eye become red and watery and sometimes produce pus. The eyelids may stick together when the person sleeps. This is due to infection with germs. Wash the eye with water, which has been boiled and cooled.

Night blindness occurs in some countries in children age 2–5. It is caused by lack of vitamin A. If not treated, the child can become permanently blind.

River blindness is a serious disease caused by tiny worms and spread by little flies which bite. The flies breed in fast-flowing rivers.

Trachoma causes sore eyes and the pain continues for a long time. Often the person becomes blind. It can be treated with the right ointment. It is a virus disease which is spread by flies and by direct contact.

The ear

An enlarged section through the ear is shown below.

The outer ear collects sound waves which hit the ear drum. The ear drum vibrates. The vibrations pass along three tiny bones. These little bones transmit the vibrations to the inner ear, which contains a fluid and nerves which are sensitive to the vibrations of the fluid. The nerves are connected to the brain. The brain interprets the pattern of nerve impulses from the ear so that we 'hear'.

The ear also helps us to balance. There are three semi-circular canals which are set at right angles to each other. They contain fluid which moves when the head moves. There are nerves in the walls of the canal which are sensitive to movement of the fluid. These nerves carry impulses to the brain and thus help us to keep our balance and posture. The middle ear contains air. It is connected by the Eustachian tube to the back of the throat. You can feel it 'popping' open as the air goes in when you swallow. This keeps the air pressure on the two sides of the eardrum the same. Sometimes infections from the throat can pass up the Eustachian tube.

The nose

The nose is part of our breathing system. When we breathe through the nose, air is warmed there before entering the lungs. Small hairs in the nose trap dust particles so that the air is also cleaned. When we breathe in, the air passes through passages (the nasal cavities) in the head. These are lined with a thin moist membrane called the mucous membrane. In this membrane are nerve cells which are sensitive to particles and droplets of substances which may be in the air. This helps to give rise to the sensation of smell. When we eat, we smell the food which is in the mouth. In this case, smell is part of taste. If we have a bad cold which blocks the nose, we cannot smell. The sense of taste is also affected.

Feet

At birth, the bones in a baby's feet are soft. They finally become hard (ossified) when the person is about 18 or 20. If a child wears shoes that are too small, the feet can become deformed (wrong shape). As children grow older, their feet change in shape as well as size. Thus, adult's shoes are not suitable for children.

Children should learn to keep their feet clean and dry. In some cases, it is important that children wear shoes because of the possibility of hookworm infection. The baby hookworms enter through the feet. Eventually they attach themselves to the wall of the gut (see chapter 5). The worms lay eggs which leave the body in the person's stools. Hookworm can cause severe weakness in children.

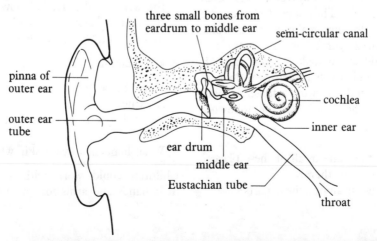

three small bones from eardrum to middle ear

semi-circular canal

pinna of outer ear

outer ear tube

cochlea

inner ear

ear drum

middle ear

Eustachian tube

throat

Some Teaching Suggestions

We need to teach children to care for their bodies. To do this, they have to understand something about them. Encourage children to be proud of having clean bodies and being attractive. This is an important part of health education. In the primary school, you can help children to develop good habits and attitudes. Remember that by the end of the primary school, many children will reach puberty with all its problems.

The skin

So far as a clean body is concerned, the skin is obviously the most important organ. We need to bathe and wash our skin to keep it clean. This removes outside dirt, dead cells, stale sweat and oil. If we do not wash, these waste secretions begin to smell and to make our clothes smell. It is important to keep skin dry as well as clean. In hot climates, we sweat more. This makes it all the more difficult to keep skin dry. If there are breaks in the skin, germs can enter. Some parasites, such as hookworm, can enter the skin even if there is no break. At puberty, the sweat glands in some areas of the body develop very rapidly. Moist, warm parts of the body should be washed more often. It is particularly important for girls to wash more carefully during menstruation. Adolescent boys and girls often get spots on their face. They should not squeeze the spots. If they do, they make the spots worse and they can squeeze germs into the body.

Encourage children to look at their skin. If available, they could use hand lenses to look at the palm of the hand, an arm, a finger, a nail, hair, the sole of the foot. Ask the following questions:

- Is the surface the same in all of these places?
- What differences are there?
- Does hair grow on any of these parts?

- Is the skin harder, thicker or thinner in some places than others?
- Is the skin always the same colour?

What does skin do?

The following are some suggestions for work with children:

- Children could list and describe the coverings of animals such as hide, scales, fur, feathers, hair, wool etc. Can they make a collection for the discovery table? How do these coverings keep the animal warm and dry? How does the human skin do this?
- If a thermometer is available, let children find out the normal body temperature. Is it the same for all children? With a clinical thermometer, you should turn it until you can see the silver line. The temperature is the place where the silver line stops.

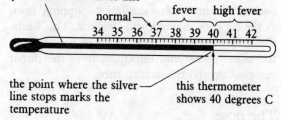

turn the thermometer until you can see the silver line

normal — fever — high fever
34 35 36 37 38 39 40 41 42

the point where the silver line stops marks the temperature

this thermometer shows 40 degrees C

Before use, clean the thermometer well with soap and water. Shake it hard with a snap of the wrist until it reads below 36°C. Put it in the mouth below a person's tongue with the mouth shut. Wash the thermometer after use.

Ask the children:

- Does the body temperature ever change and if so, when?
- What happens to your skin when you get cold?
- What happens to your skin when you get hot?

Children could work with a partner to test their hands and arms for touch sensitivity.

- One child closes his eyes. The other touches the skin gently with a sharp pencil or pin. Can he feel it? Touch other places. Which parts of the skin are most sensitive? This experiment works even better if two pencils are used. Sometimes the prick feels like one point, sometimes like two. Can the child who is being touched distinguish if one or two pencils are being used? The finger tips, for example, are much more sensitive than the skin of the back. Children could try the activity suggested on page 14 (Feeling the textures of different objects).

Looking after skin

Either through planned lessons or at appropriate times, we need to make sure that children understand why we should wash:

Why should we wash? To remove: dirt and grease dead skin germs	If we don't wash The result is: smell clogged pores spoiled clothes skin disease like scabies
Everyday washing hands, face, neck, ears between legs genital organs under arms feet	**Take particular care** before meals after going to the lavatory during menstruation after activity

Remember what we have said about changes in the skin during adolescence. Help children to understand what causes spots and pimples. Stress the need to clean regularly with soap and water. Reassure them that spots are common in adolescence.

Ringworm of the scalp and body is quite common, especially when children do not wash frequently.

Looking after hair

Care of hair is important for your personal appearance. What hair styles do children in your class have? (See photographs on page 31.)

Hair should be kept clean. It should be regularly washed, brushed and combed. It should also be checked for lice.

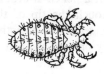

Lice cause itching and sometimes skin infections. You can use a special shampoo to treat lice. Nits, which are the eggs of lice, cement themselves to the hair. They can be removed by combing with a fine toothcomb. If children have lice, teach them to put their bedding out in the sun. Help children to think about hair care. For instance, in towns children will probably see many advertisements for shampoo. Are shampoos essential?

Looking after nails

Let children examine their nails and those of their friends. Finger nails should be cut rounded, and toe nails cut straight. Show children how to cut their nails. Explain that it is important to clean out the dirt from under nails.

The eye

It is obvious to children that our eyes are very precious. We have to look after them. But eyes are not like skin or teeth. We don't have to wash them or clean them. If they are functioning satisfactorily, we should leave them alone.

Let children compare their eyes with those of animals. Ask questions like these:

- How are the eyes of animals similar to ours?
- How are they different?
- Why do we have two eyes?

27

- Why are our eyes at the front of our heads? (The position of our eyes enables us to judge distances accurately. It is much more difficult to judge distance with only one eye.)

Let children try this experiment:

- They hold out a pencil at arm's length. Then they try to touch the tip of the pencil with their index finger (a) when both eyes are open (b) when only one eye is open.

Other questions you could ask are:
- What is the function of our eyebrows and lashes and of eyesockets and eyelids?
- Would it be useful to have eyes in the backs of our heads? Or on our finger tips?
- How do eyes show what we are feeling? Can children draw sad, frightened or happy eyes?

Let children look into their partner's eyes.
- Shine a torch into the eye (or look at a bright light). What happens? Cover the eyes for a few minutes. Now open them. What has happened?
- Make a class book about eyes. Different children could contribute to different parts of the book. Or children could work in groups.

Looking after eyes

On page 24, we considered some eye problems. Help children to understand these and to understand why some children need to wear spectacles. Here are a few important points:

- avoid rubbing the eyes
- don't look directly at the sun
- try to have good light when reading books
- wear spectacles if needed
- protect the eyes from dust and chippings
- take care near thorn bushes
- never poke sticks or pointed objects at the faces of other children

(See also page 187 for how to test the eyesight of children.)

The ear

The ears are important for communication. Children can easily understand this. It is less easy for them to understand that the ear is a balance organ (see page 25).

- Get a child to turn round and round quickly. What happens? What does he see?
- Get children to find our how good their hearing is. Hold up a watch near the ear. How far away can they take it and still hear it ticking? Record the distance. Is it the same for the other ear? How do they compare with their group or class? If no watch is available, can children think of other quiet sounds? Can they whisper to each other? How do they make sure that whispers are of the same loudness?
- Why do we need two ears? Blindfold a child and make a noise. For example, snap a finger

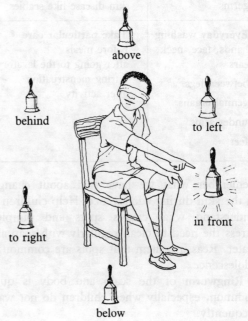

above

behind

to left

to right

in front

below

28

or ring a bell. Can the child point out from where he thinks the noise is coming? Block up one ear. Does this make it easier or more difficult to say from where the sound is coming? Ask him to keep his head still. Does this make it even more difficult?

- Children could list animals which can hear very well. Discuss the advantages of sensitive hearing with them. These are: protection (it is important that animals can detect predators); communication; and in the case of the bat, direction finding. (Bats cannot see well. Instead they make high pitched squeaks which bounce off objects and come back to their big ears. It is a kind of radar mechanism.)
- Ask children why we need ears. Can children list dangerous sounds and happy sounds? Can they list sounds which they hear on their way to school? Can they list sounds which they hear near their homes or sounds in the morning and in the evening?

Looking after ears

Ears should be kept dry and clean. Children should understand that they should not poke hard objects into their ears. It is not necessary to clean inside the ear. Wax falls out by itself. It has a job to do – to catch and carry out dust.

The nose

Help children to understand that the nose is part of the breathing system (see page 37). The nose allows us to smell. Ask the children:

- Why do we need the sense of smell?
- What is the advantage for us?
  (It helps us to detect danger, for example, the smell of burning. It also gives us pleasure such as the smell of food or smell of flowers and scent.)
- What animals have a good sense of smell?
- What is the advantage for them?

Make up some smelling boxes. For example,

put strongly smelling things into labelled matchboxes. You could use coffee, paint, orange juice, mouldy food, onion, curry powder, local smelly fruits and seeds. (**Do not use dangerous substances like petrol or insecticides.**)

- Can the children say what the smells are?
- Can they make up their own smelling boxes?

Find out what smells children like most (or least). Can they make a table or bar chart to show this information?

Looking after the nose

Encourage children to cover their mouths and noses when they cough or sneeze. Tell them to blow their nose gently.

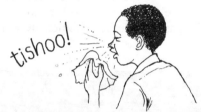

'Coughs and sneezes spread diseases!'

If you blow your nose too hard, infection can spread back up to the ear. It is better to blow one nostril at a time. Explain to the children how to stop nose bleeds. (You pinch below the bridge of the nose and tip the head forwards.)

Clothes and shoes

Why do we wear clothes? Discuss this point with children. One of the most important reasons is that clothes help us to keep warm in cold weather. If we are cold, we put on more clothes. If we are hot, we take them off. In hot countries, it is important to wear cool, suitable clothing. Three points about clothes are:

- Cotton materials are best. Cotton absorbs sweat and allows it to evaporate. The artificial fibres (like nylon and terylene) are not so comfortable. They also become smelly more quickly.

- Light, whitish colours reflect the sun and are cooler. Dark materials absorb the heat.
- Clothes should be loose and open.

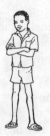

Discuss these ideas with children. Do they suggest that we also wear clothes to look attractive? Discuss the clothes traditionally worn in your area.

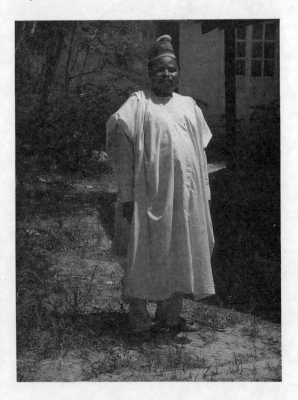

Here are some activities that you could do with the children:

- Can the children make a collection of local clothes?
- Can they obtain pictures of clothing from other parts of the world?
- What sort of hats or other headresses are worn? Are they traditional? Do they have religious significance? What clothes are worn for special occasions? (For example at festivals, weddings or parties.) Why do some people wear uniforms?
- If you take your children on a visit to the market, let them visit the tailor. Invite a tailor to your school. Perhaps he could explain to the children how he makes clothes. Let him give a demonstration if possible so that the children can ask questions.
- Can the children make a collection of the different materials used to make clothes?

Many children in hot countries do not wear shoes. Or they wear simple plastic 'flip-flops.' Shoes for children are expensive. Their feet are continually growing so that shoes often have to be renewed. As a teacher, you need to be aware of these problems. For health reasons, children should wear shoes if possible. Teach children to wash the feet carefully every day with soap and water. Otherwise, the feet should be kept dry.

Looking after clothes
Clothes should be washed often, especially underclothes and socks. Remember that for some children and families, soap or washing powder may be expensive.
Ask the children:

- Who washes their clothes?
- Do they help their mothers?
- Where are clothes washed?
- Is lack of water a problem?

Grooming

You can help children to bring together the ideas suggested so far in this chapter. Perhaps they could make up a checklist for their own grooming. Let them talk with you about what they actually do. Is this the same as what they ought to do? Why is there a difference between the two? Remember what we said at the beginning of this chapter. It is important that we are realistic in our expectations of children. The checklist might look something like this:

Daily	Weekly	Regularly
clean nails	wash hair	cut hair
brush or comb hair	cut finger nails	cut toe nails
clean teeth	wash clothes	
wash hands		
(several times a day)		
wash body		

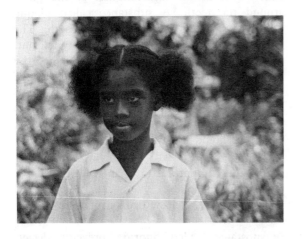
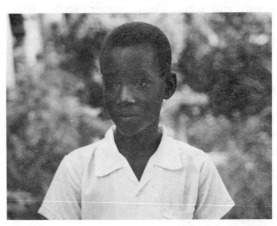
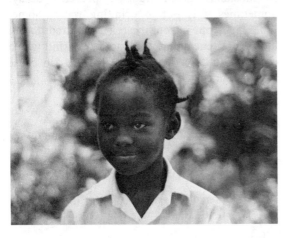
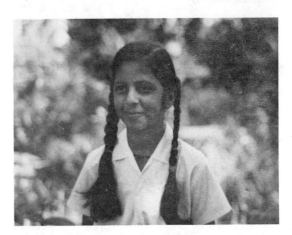

Hair! Look after it!

Useful Background Knowledge

Teeth

Teeth and what they do

When we are born, the teeth are not visible. However, they are already there in the upper and lower jaw bones. At about 3–4 months, the first teeth (or milk teeth) begin to push through the gums. By two years most children have about twenty milk teeth. The permanent teeth start to appear at about the age of six and they push out the milk teeth. By the time you are an adult, you will have thirty two permanent teeth.

The milk and permanent teeth are arranged as shown below.

The **incisors** are cutting teeth. The **canines** are for tearing. The **molars** are for grinding. So, the front teeth are for biting and the back ones are for chewing.

Good teeth allow us to:

- eat a variety of foods
- look attractive
- speak clearly

What can go wrong?

Teeth can **decay** (become rotten). Certain foods, especially sugar, sweets, biscuits and cake, can cause the process of decay. This happens when the food is left on the teeth. Germs eat the sugar and make an acid which attacks the tooth. The tooth becomes brown. Later a hole appears. The hole may be small at first. But it gradually gets bigger. If the hole is not filled, the person suffers from toothache. The tooth then becomes so rotten that it breaks off. Really rotten teeth can affect the health of the rest of our body.

Another important problem is **periodontal disease**. This means inflammation of the gums around the teeth. A substance called **plaque** builds up around the base of the tooth. The gums become inflamed. The tooth may fall out. Teach children that it can be prevented by brushing near to the base of teeth to remove plaque.

Help children to understand these ideas. Help them to prevent decay and periodontal disease. Children should learn two key points:

- it is most important to clean teeth to remove sugar and plaque
- sweet foods and fizzy drinks rot teeth

A substance called **fluoride** prevents decay. Sometimes it is put in drinking water. Sometimes, it is put in toothpaste. If children do use toothpaste, encourage them to buy a kind which contains fluoride. Too much fluoride can cause brown stained teeth.

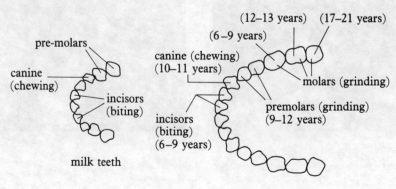

milk teeth

permanent teeth

Some Teaching Suggestions

Looking at teeth

Children could look at teeth of younger brothers and sisters, older children, babies, other pupils in their own class and adults. Here are some suggestions:

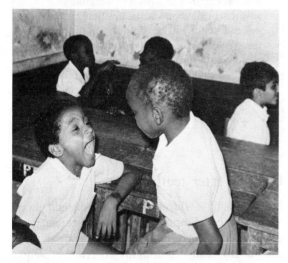

Get children to count the number of teeth in a person's mouth. Ask the children:

- Does everyone have the same number?
- What is the maximum number of teeth in a mouth?
- How many teeth do babies have?
- Do all the teeth look the same?
- Why do we have different teeth?

Discuss the children's observations with them. Can they make drawings to show the arrangement of teeth in the mouth?

- When children's milk teeth fall out, encourage them to bring them to school. Discuss with children why teeth are important. What is it like to have no teeth? What problems does a person with no teeth have?

Can the children find skulls from dead animals? Ask the children:

- Are animal teeth different from ours?
- How are they different?
- Why are they different?

You could discuss with children the teeth of familiar animals. For example, the dog is a meat eater (a carnivore). It has different teeth from a cow which eats grass (a herbivore).

Explain to children that we have two sets of teeth. Remind them that their permanent teeth are their last.

Do any of the children have younger brothers and sisters? Ask the children:

- Are they bottle-fed?
- Do any of them suck continually on a bottle?

Explain to the children that this is very bad for a young child's teeth. The sugar in the liquid quickly rots their teeth.

In looking at other children's teeth ask if any of them had holes. Ask the children:

- What do the holes look like?
- Do any have fillings?
- What do the fillings look like?
- Which teeth usually have fillings?

Explain to children about the effects of sweet foods and fizzy drinks.

- Get two milk teeth. Drop one into water and one into a bottled fizzy drink. Leave them for a few days. Then take them out and observe them. You will find that the tooth in the water stays healthy. But the tooth in the fizzy drink becomes soft. You can scrape some of it off. (Don't tell the children what they will see. Do the experiment and let the children observe for themselves.)

Children should go to a dentist or dental worker if they have holes in their teeth. Obviously this is not possible everywhere.

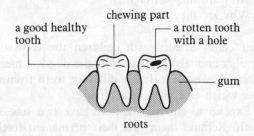

a good healthy tooth

chewing part

a rotten tooth with a hole

gum

roots

A play

The children could do a play or make a puppet theatre. Suggestions for the characters are as follows:

Jimmy Germ	— a bad man
Simon Sugar	— a bad man who rots teeth ('a rotter')
Sammy Molar	— a good but rather stupid man
Mr Dental Worker \ Mrs Brushstick /	— two good helpful people who stop Jimmy Germ and Simon Sugar from attacking Sammy Molar

The plot might be something like this. You and the children could develop it as you like. For example, you could involve more of the children by letting them be 'germs' or 'sugar'.

1 Sammy Molar tells Mr Dental Worker what it is like to be a tooth. He says how frightened he is of Jimmy Germ and Simon Sugar.
2 Jimmy Germ and Simon Sugar appear and say how they plan to rot Sammy Molar.
3 Mr Dental Worker and Mrs Brushstick talk about protecting Sammy Molar.
4 Sammy Molar gets covered in sweet food by Simon Sugar. Jimmy Germ and Simon Sugar jump on Sammy Molar who starts to go bad. He calls for help. Mrs Brushstick appears and pushes off Jimmy Germ and Simon Sugar.

5 Sammy Molar describes his lucky escape to Mr Dental Worker. He explains the importance of not eating too much sweet food and cleaning the teeth.

A radio broadcast and a comic strip

- Ask the children to write a two-minute advertisement about dental health. Let them pretend that it will be broadcast on the radio. If there is a tape recorder available, the children could record the advertisement.
- Children could make up a comic strip about good care of the teeth. Let them pretend that it is for a children's newspaper or magazine.

Looking after teeth

Discuss with children how they should keep teeth clean. Emphasise the importance of brushing them regularly. Clean them at least once a day really thoroughly to remove plaque and sugar. Give them an extra clean after eating food with sugar in it.

- Children could make chew sticks. They look like this:

use the twig of a tree

chew on this end and use the fibres as a brush

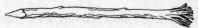

Find the twig of a suitable tree. Often local people know a good tree. Chew on the end and use the fibres as a brush. Sharpen the other end to a point. With this, the food can be removed from between the teeth. Of course, children can use toothbrushes if they have them.

- Teach them how to make tooth powder. Mix salt and bicarbonate of soda in equal amounts:

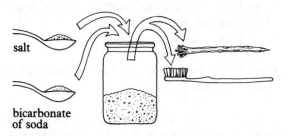

salt

bicarbonate of soda

If no bicarbonate of soda is available, salt by itself can be used. Wet the brush before use so that the powder sticks to it.

- Show children how to brush their teeth. The brush should clean all the surfaces of the teeth including the inner surfaces. It is best to brush up and down, to flick out the food between the teeth. Brush the biting surfaces with a backwards and forwards scrubbing movement. Clean near to the gums.

Do's and Don'ts for teeth and gums

Help children make up a checklist for looking after teeth and gums. Perhaps it might look like the one below.

The mouth and tongue

When teaching about teeth, don't forget the mouth and tongue.

Ask the children:
- What does the mouth look like?
- What can we do with our mouths? (lick, whistle, chew, spit, kiss, smile etc.)
- How do we use our mouths to demonstrate our moods, such as happiness, anger or sadness?
- What does the tongue do?

The tongue has the following functions:

- it helps us to chew
- it moves food around the mouth
- it is necessary for speech
- it tastes food (there are four taste areas on the tongue: sweet, salt, sour, bitter)

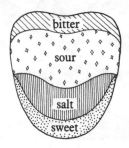

Can the children map these areas? Use salt, sugar, lemon juice, vinegar etc. Put a drop of each on different parts of the tongue. Use a straw or clean stick. What part does the nose play in taste? Get children to hold their nose when they try this experiment. (Remember what we said about safety in chapter 2. Children should do experiments on tasting only under supervision.)

Do	Don't
• brush teeth every day	• let teeth rot
• brush teeth before going to bed	• forget to brush teeth
• eat healthy foods	• use broken brick, charcoal or other hard materials for cleaning teeth
• teach younger brothers and sisters to brush their teeth.	• drink fizzy drinks
• have a brush or brushstick for each person in the family . . . and so on	• eat many sweets and sugar
	• use one brush for everyone in the family . . . and so on

Useful background knowledge

Healthy living

Exercise, rest and recreation are essential for healthy lives. They are necessary for our **physical** health and for our **mental** health.

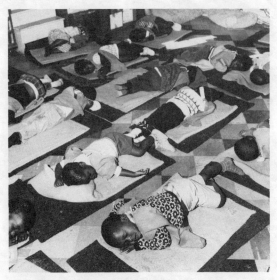

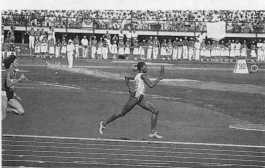

What do we know about exercise and the body's need for rest?

- we know that the body needs frequent and vigorous exercise: it must be vigorous enough to change the pulse and breathing rates

- we know that joints should be exercised to keep them flexible
- we know that muscles grow stronger with use and weaker with lack of use
- we know that, without sleep, the body rapidly becomes exhausted
- we know that a physically healthy body makes us feel good

Perhaps children will learn some of these ideas in physical education lessons. It is important that they understand that exercise, rest and sleep are essential to keep physically and mentally fit.

Exercise

During exercise:

- the nerves stimulate muscles which contract and relax
- the muscles enable the body to move
- the muscles need more fuel (from food) and oxygen (from air)
- the muscles produce carbon dioxide, water and heat
- the heart pumps faster to provide more fuel and oxygen to the muscles and remove waste products
- the lungs work harder to provide more oxygen and remove the carbon dioxide

As waste products build up, the body feels fatigued. When exercise stops, the heart and lungs continue to work faster to restore the balance of fuel, oxygen and waste.
Exercise keeps the body in good working order in the following ways:

- it keeps joints flexible
- it makes muscles strong
- it keeps weight down
- it keeps our heart and blood vessels in good order

- it makes the body feel tired so that we sleep better
- it generally makes us feel fit and well

In Africa and Asia, many children get plenty of exercise. They may have to walk a long way to school. They may have to work at home. Always remember this when you are teaching about exercise.

Rest and sleep

The body is functioning all the time, even when we are resting or sleeping. The cells of the body need a continuous supply of oxygen and fuel. Waste products such as carbon dioxide and water must be continually removed. During rest or sleep, the cells are fed and become ready for further activity. We lose our sense of fatigue.

During sleep a number of changes take place in the body:

- the pulse rate falls
- body temperature drops
- muscles relax
- blood pressure falls
- we dream

In recent years, scientists have learnt a lot about sleep. We now know that there are different levels of sleep. The brain continues to work when we are asleep but its electrical patterns change throughout the night. Sometimes the eyes move quickly from side to side. These are called Rapid Eye Movements (REMs for short). They happen when we are in a shallow period of sleep and when we are dreaming. Dreaming is very important. If people are continually woken up in REM periods, they feel as though they have had no sleep. Everyone dreams. However, we only tend to remember dreams when we are woken up during a period of shallow sleep.

How much sleep?

Some books recommend that children of a particular age require a specific amount of sleep. Obviously, babies need more sleep than children and children need more sleep than adults. But we cannot make hard and fast rules about this. All individuals are different. But we should try to make sure that children do not feel exhausted when they start school. Encourage children to learn about their own sleep patterns. It is much better if they have a regular routine. Remember that, in some places, children have to walk a long way to and from school. Remember also that some children may have to help their parents at home with a farm or garden. If they share a room, other people may keep them awake at night.

The lungs and breathing

Our bodies are made up of millions of cells. There are many different kinds of cells. Here are a few examples:

- muscle cells
- nerve cells
- liver cells
- bone cells
- blood cells . . . and so on

In order to stay alive and do its job, a cell needs oxygen and food. Consider a muscle cell. It receives oxygen and food through the blood. It releases the energy in the food and contracts. The cell becomes hotter and it produces certain waste products. These include carbon dioxide and water.

The waste products are normally carried away by the blood. However, during vigorous exercise the blood cannot move them away fast enough. The muscles feel tired or painful. They have to rest.

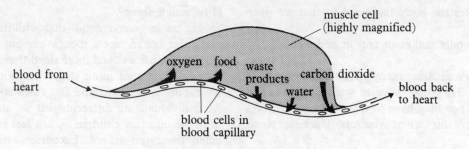

oxygen food waste products carbon dioxide water

muscle cell (highly magnified)

blood from heart

blood back to heart

blood cells in blood capillary

How do the cells get oxygen?

As we have seen, all the cells of the body need oxygen. Oxygen is a gas. It is part of the air (about ⅕th by volume). Air passes into the lungs. The oxygen from the air passes into the blood. The blood is pumped around the body and delivers the oxygen to the cells.

The lungs

When we breathe in, air passes down the windpipe (trachea) into smaller and smaller pipes into the lungs.

The small pipes end in tiny air sacs. Blood comes to and from these air sacs in very small blood vessels.

The oxygen from the air passes into the blood. The carbon dioxide in the blood passes into the air in the lungs which is breathed out (see below and opposite page right).

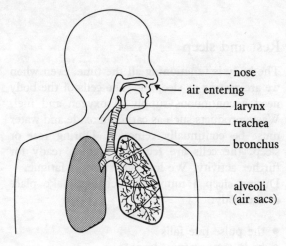

nose
air entering
larynx
trachea
bronchus
alveoli (air sacs)

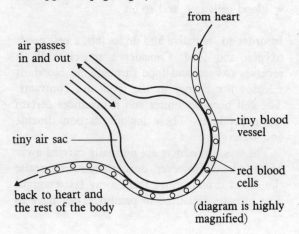

from heart

air passes in and out

tiny air sac

tiny blood vessel

red blood cells

back to heart and the rest of the body

(diagram is highly magnified)

Breathing

How does the air get in and out of our lungs? First, the muscles between the ribs contract. The ribs move upwards and outwards. Secondly, a big muscle – the diaphragm – which is just above the stomach, contracts and moves downwards. The result is that air now passes into the lungs. The rib muscles and diaphragm then relax. The lungs are elastic so they contract and squeeze out the air. In this way we breathe out.

When we take exercise, the muscles need more oxygen, so the lungs have to work harder. They have to bring in more oxygen and take away more carbon dioxide. We thus have to breathe more quickly. We don't have to 'think' about this. The body does it automatically. There is, in fact, a special part of the brain which controls the rate of breathing.

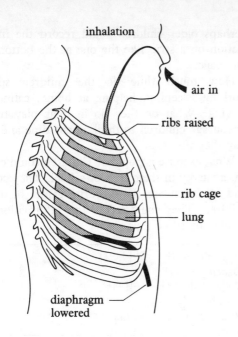

inhalation

air in

ribs raised

rib cage

lung

diaphragm
lowered

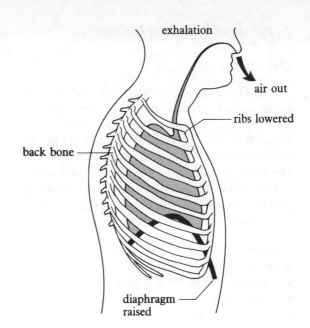

exhalation

air out

ribs lowered

back bone

diaphragm
raised

The heart and circulation

The heart pumps the blood around the body. You can think of it as two pumps, side by side, which work like this:

- One pump receives blood containing carbon dioxide. This blood comes from the body. This pump pumps the blood to the lungs. There, the blood gives up its carbon dioxide which is breathed out. The blood takes up fresh oxygen from the air in the lungs.
- The other pump receives the blood which has absorbed oxygen from the air. It pumps this at high pressure to the rest of the body.

Arteries are blood vessels taking blood away from the heart. They have thick walls.

Veins bring blood back to the heart. They have thin walls. They have valves in them to stop the blood from flowing backwards.

The **heart beat** (or pulse) is about 130 beats per minute for a new-born baby, and about 70 for adults. For primary school children, it may be 80–100 beats per minute. When we exercise,

the heart beats faster. This is so that our muscles can get more oxygen and fuel and waste products can be taken away more quickly. The high pulse rate continues after exercise until the proper balance in the body has been restored.

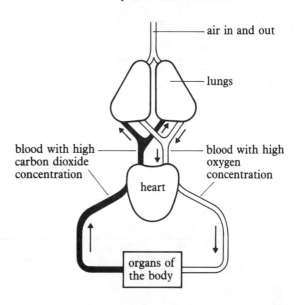

air in and out

lungs

blood with high
carbon dioxide
concentration

blood with high
oxygen
concentration

heart

organs of
the body

Some Teaching Suggestions

Organising our time

The day has twenty four hours only and we have to do certain essential things. For example, we have to eat, sleep and work. We have to get to and from school. We have only a little time for leisure activities. How do we use this time? How can we help children to use it wisely and well?

Let children consider how they spend a normal day during term time. Help them to think about their various activities such as:

- sleeping
- eating
- travelling to and from school
- school work
- helping at home
- playing

How much time do they spend on these activities? Younger children could make a diagram to summarise the information, perhaps like this:

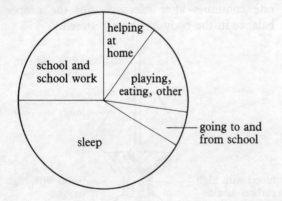

Perhaps older children could record the information on a strip like the one at the bottom of this page.

How much time do the children spend working, sleeping, helping at home, eating or playing? What do they do in their play time? Encourage children to think about time and the way they use it.

What exercise is popular? Children could carry out a survey in their class or school. They could find out what are the favourite games of other children. They could record this information on a tally chart like this:

Football	++++ ++++ |||
Dancing	++++	
Volley Ball	++++ ++++
Walking	++++
Running	++++ ++++	

They could convert the information to a bar chart by getting information from other classes. They could try to find out whether girls have different preferences from boys. If the school has a cassette tape recorder, you or the children could record interviews. The interview could be with older or younger children or adults. Questions might include:

- What is your favourite exercise?
- How do you take most exercise?
- Which sportsman or woman do you admire most?

You or the children could collect pictures from newspapers or magazines of sportsmen and

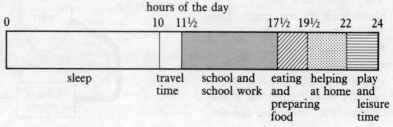

women and make a display. Can you find photographs of any nationally known ones?

The children could do their own drawings of people playing sports and put them on the display. Pin or stick the pictures to cardboard. Put the display on the classroom wall.

How do we move around?

Below are some questions which you might use with children. Perhaps you could ask these questions to start a discussion with children, or use them for their homework, or put them on work cards:

- How many ways of moving around can you think of?
- How many of these ways use muscle power?
- What other methods do we use to move around?
- What advantages have these methods brought us?
- What disadvantages do these methods have?

Make a large map of the area around your school. Mark the homes of all the children in your class. You could use a colour code or symbols. How do the children come to school? (Remember that this is likely to vary according to whether the school is in the town or country.) Walking, cycling and bus are probably the most common methods. Where are the danger places for children when coming to school? Mark them on the map. (See 'Safety First' chapter 6.)

What happens when we take exercise?

Children could take the following measurements before and after vigorous exercise:

- pulse rate (show children how to take the pulse by resting the finger tips on the wrist in the position shown here)

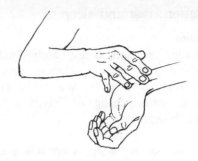

- breathing rate
- temperature (if a thermometer is available)

The exercise might be running around the school field several times. Or it could be stepping on and off a chair or stool. Or whatever you or the children suggest. Repeat the experiment and record the results in the form of a bar chart. Ask the following questions:

- How long does it take for the heart and breathing rates to return to normal?
- Does it take the same time for all children and, if not, why not?

Let children make a poster showing the effects of exercise.

Ask the children:

- How do you feel after taking exercise?
- How do you feel after taking too much exercise?
- Why do we sweat if we take a lot of exercise?
- Why should we wash after sweating?

Can children explain why heart and breathing rates increase after exercise? Use the background information on pages 38 and 39. Perhaps the children could make a class book about the effects of exercise on the body. You could relate this work to your science lessons.

Relaxation, rest and sleep

Relaxation

Is relaxation the same as rest? Help children to understand that relaxation may sometimes involve vigorous exercise. We could say that relaxation means a change of activity.
Ask the children:

- Can you go on taking vigorous exercise for several hours?
- How do you know when to stop?

Time the children on a particular task (running 100 m for example). How long does it take? Try again: How long does it take this time? Do the same again. What effect does this have?

Ask the children:

- What do you like doing when you are physically tired. What do you like to do when you are mentally tired?
- How do you like to relax?
- Do you have to do nothing in order to relax?

Rest

When we rest, we reduce the amount of physical or mental activity going on in the body. This is different from relaxation.
Ask the children:

- What do you find restful?

- If you find music restful, is all music restful?
- Does everyone find the same music restful?
- What other sounds are restful and what are not restful?
- Are all colours restful and does everyone find the same colours restful?
- Can you draw restful pictures?

Sleep

Talk to the children about sleep. (See background information p. 37.) Find out if children dream. What do they say about their dreams? Perhaps they could watch their younger brothers and sisters who are asleep. How much sleep do the children get? Do they all sleep the same amount? Emphasise the importance of plenty of sleep.

They could find out the sleep periods of
- 5-year-olds
- 10-year-olds
- 15-year-olds

They could compare these with the average sleep periods of their own class.

Can they make a poster advertising the effects of sleep or the bad effects of no sleep? Can they advertise the benefits of getting up early in the mornings?

Chapter Three

Ourselves and Others

Useful Background Knowledge

Family, school, community

We are human beings. We live together on a small planet called earth. By the year 2 000 AD, there will be more than 6 000 million people on earth. We have to feed and clothe ourselves. We have to provide schools, hospitals, clean water and fuel. We are using up coal, oil and vital minerals at a frightening rate. We have terrible weapons which could destroy the human race. So it is important that we learn to live with each other. We are dependent upon other people. Other people are dependent upon us.

The last two chapters were about ourselves and how to look after ourselves. This chapter is about our relationships with other people. You will find that many of the ideas in the later pages of this book are also relevant here.

There are many ways in which we learn about other people. Most important is the family.

In the family, we learn:

- to share happiness and sorrow with others
- about our feelings of love and hate for others
- about other people's needs and wants
- about other people's moods and personalities
- about the ways in which we can help or hurt them

Whether the family is small or large, it contains the people who are usually closest to us. From these people, we learn much of our behaviour. Through our family, we learn what other people are like.

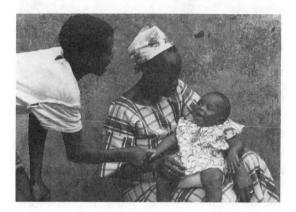

When we go to school we meet a much wider circle of people. We meet children who come from homes which are different from ours. We meet adults called **teachers**. We behave differently to our teachers than to our parents. They behave differently to us. For most of us, school is the first organised institution which we enter. It is a place with rules and customs. It has a timetable. It is a place to which our parents do not often come. In a school, children learn about other people. It can be a happy or an unhappy place. It can be a caring or an uncaring place. It can be a place where children learn good attitudes and habits or the opposite. Which it is, depends very largely on teachers. The teacher's role is much more than just teaching knowledge and skills.

We also learn about other people from our community. This may be a village or a town. We may meet many people other than our family or just a few. Although these people may not be as close to us as our parents, brothers and sisters, they are **people**. They react to us. We react to them. We learn that such people have certain roles such as shopkeepers, policemen, health workers, mechanics, headmen of the villages.

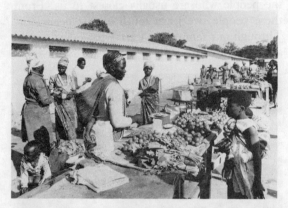

In the family, school and community, we also learn about our role as a boy or a girl. Every society gives different roles to girls and boys, women and men. We learn that boys and girls dress differently, that their bodies are different.

When they grow up they tend to have different jobs. Some people think that, in the past, these differences have been over-emphasised. After all, many girls enjoy doing things which are meant to be boys' activities. Many boys enjoy doing things which are meant to be girls' activities.

Between the ages of about eleven and fifteen, boys and girls become sexually mature. This time is called **puberty**. Boys and girls of this age become interested in people of the opposite sex. At this time, the feeling of sexual attraction in us is often very strong. We have to learn how to cope with these strong feelings. We have to remember that people of the opposite sex are still **people**. They have feelings and opinions just like we do.

So, from our family, school and community, we learn how to live with other people. As a young baby or child, we see ourselves as the centre of our world. Gradually we learn that other people have feelings, problems, needs, desires and opinions. School is only one place where this learning takes place. But, as a teacher, you have the opportunity to encourage it. Of course, it is not only in health education that such opportunities arise. In social studies, moral, religious and physical education, and in extra-curricular activities such as scouting, useful incidents and issues will occur. It is important to learn how to use these opportunities.

Some Teaching Suggestions

Work with younger children

There is much work which you would normally do with older children which you could perhaps extend to younger children. Here are some ideas:

What is mine? What is ours?
Help children to understand that some things belong only to them (for example, their clothes or their schoolbags). Ask them to make a list of things which belong to them and to others. Discuss with them for example:
- our teacher
- our desks
- our books
- our classroom

What does it mean when we talk about 'our classroom'? It means that we **share** the classroom with others. We all have responsibility for it. We can keep it clean or leave it dirty. Get the children to discuss why it matters to keep the classroom clean and tidy.

Do we help each other?
You could draw a picture of two children fighting on the board and ask the children to make up a story about this.

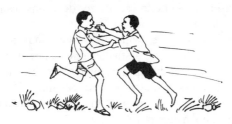

Or ask two children to come to the front of the class and argue. You could suggest a little play. The plot might be that one child thinks another has stolen his or her book. Let them imagine how they might behave. Then let them at it. Discuss with the class:
- why are the children quarrelling?

- what will happen next?
- what happened in the end?
- how could they end the quarrel happily?
- have you ever felt like them?

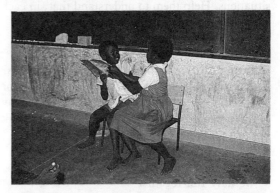

Two children acting out a role play: quarrelling over a book

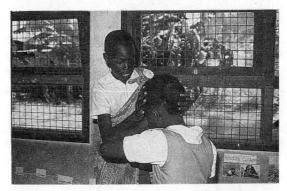

Role play: one child tells his father about the quarrel

Help children to describe quarrels which they have had. What caused them? How could they be avoided?

Children could write short stories or draw pictures to illustrate quarrels.

In what ways do we help each other? Children could act out little plays, showing for example:

- a child is hurt, she starts to cry, another child comforts her
- a child helps a blind person to cross a road
- two children teach a third how to play a game

- a child helps her mother at home
- a boy helps his father on the farm

Let children produce their own ideas for these situations. Help them to understand that, in each case, they are cooperating.

Why is my friend my friend?

Why do we like some people and not others? It is often difficult to say why, especially for children. They may want to say 'My friend is my friend because I like him.' But help them to think beyond this. For example, they might suggest:
- we like doing the same things
- we live near each other
- we have fun together
- he or she is cheerful
- he or she has a friendly family

What is a family?

What do children mean when they talk about a family? Many families in Africa and other parts of the world are very large. They may consist of parents, children, aunts, uncles, cousins and grandparents:

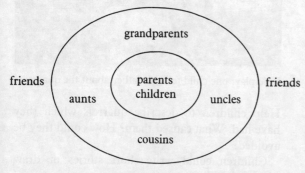

Other families are much smaller consisting only of parents and children:

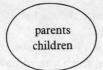

But whatever its size, we should help children to understand that a family is a fairly permanent group of people who:

- love each other
- care for each other
- share with each other
- help each other
- teach each other
- learn from each other

Help children to think where they belong in a family. Let children talk about the roles of their family members. Who does what at home? Do boys and girls, fathers and mothers do different jobs? If so, why?

Work with older children

With older children their relationships with others are increasingly important. In particular, they become more concerned about other children of the same age – their **peers**. They look for approval from their peers. They join groups with their peers and they make friends with their peers.

Making decisions

As children get older, they have to learn to make decisions. Sometimes, these decisions can be very hard.

Ask the children what they would do if they see a big boy bullying a smaller one. They may feel that they should help the smaller boy. But, if they do, they know that they may get hurt. Do they take the easy way out and do nothing? Or do they help the smaller boy?

Help children to act some little plays where decisions are hard. You might like to discuss suitable situations with your fellow students. Here are some ideas.
- One child sees another stealing something. What does she do?

- A boy is hurt in a football game. What does his friend do?
- A girl is late coming home because she has been playing with her friend. Her mother is angry? What happens?
- A boy is offered a cigarette by his friend. He does not want to smoke, but he does not want to seem like a coward. What does he do?

It is most important to discuss the play with the children so that they understand the point of it. It is important that they realise that the most difficult thing is **making the decision**.

Belonging to groups

Ask children to think about what groups they belong to. For example, they may say:
- country
- school
- family
- scouts
- church/mosque/or other religious group
- young farmers

Why do people belong to groups? What responsibilities do they have to the groups? What happens if the group expects us to do something which we know is wrong?

Friends

For older children, friends are even more important than for younger ones. Up to and past puberty, children mostly make friends with others of the same sex. (In some cultures, friends are always of the same sex.) We make friends because we share interests with them, because we need someone to talk to and to share secrets with. Children need to make friends. It helps them to understand what is involved in a relationship.

Ask children to list the qualities that they would look for in a friend of the same sex. To help them in this, ask questions such as:
- What is a friend for?
- Do you need to be able to talk to somebody?
- Do you want to share your worries and problems?
- Does the appearance of a friend matter to you?
- Do your friends have the same interests as you?

Perhaps the children could try to decide which of these qualities are most important for them. Encourage them to discuss questions such as these.

Useful Background Knowledge

Disabled people

It is not easy to define exactly what we mean by a disabled person. There are many different kinds of disability which may range from slight to very severe. However, here we consider that a disabled person is one who suffers from some defect of the **body, mind** or **senses** (usually hearing or seeing). Because of these defects, a disabled person is unable to do those things which other people of their age normally can do. They may behave strangely or have difficulty in learning, communicating, moving about, looking after themselves, having a job or living in the community. About eight or nine people in every hundred are disabled to a greater or lesser extent.

The effect of a disability on people depends on their attitudes to the disability. It also depends on the attitudes of the people around them: family, friends, teachers, community. For example, one child with a paralysed leg may be miserable and unhappy. But another child with a similar condition may be cheerful and able to do almost everything which other children can do.

Disabled people – like other people – want to be needed and loved. They want to be able to do a useful job of work. Children need to participate wherever possible in the games and activities of their friends. Often, disabled people can do certain things better than other people. For example, a blind person may have particularly sensitive hearing. A person who cannot walk may have very strong hands. It is important for them to feel that there are some things which they are good at and can do well. We can give them opportunities to help by using their particular strengths and talents.

Different kinds of disability

Physical

Physically disabled people have difficulty in moving. They may not be able to move their arms or legs properly. They may have difficulty in feeding or looking after themselves. Their legs may be weak. They may have difficulty in walking around. They may find it difficult to sit up or to hold up their heads. They may have other disabilities also. For example, they may not be able to speak or hear properly. Physically disabled children should be encouraged to come to school. They may have to use sticks, crutches, walking frames or wheelchairs. They may not be able to sit up like other children. They may need to lie down.

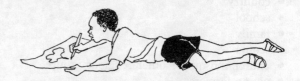

Some children may find it difficult to write. They may find it easier to write if a pencil is made thicker by wrapping a cloth around it (see also the diagram on page 57). Older children or volunteers can help these children to benefit from school. Remember that they can learn to do many things for themselves. They can often learn to enjoy life as much as other people and do a job.

Sensory

Deafness and blindness (or bad eyesight) are the most important sensory disabilities.

People may be born without sight or become blind later because of illness. They can learn to do many things for themselves by using their other senses more, especially touch and hearing. Older children can often help blind children by reading books to them and looking after them.

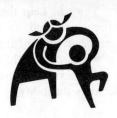

Similarly, people may be unable to hear from birth or may become deaf later in life. Because they cannot hear, many deaf people have difficulty in speaking or expressing themselves. The main problem, therefore, for deaf people is that they cannot communicate well with other people. However, they can learn to communicate in other ways. They can learn to use sign language, lip reading, body langugue, picture messages and can learn to read. They can also learn to speak. As teachers, we can encourage them in all these ways. Children who are extremely deaf should, if possible, go to a special school.

Mental

Some people may have brains which do not function well. They find it difficult to learn and understand things. They may behave strangely. In severe cases, they may not know who they are, understand what other people are saying or know how to take care of themselves. Some children who are mentally handicapped (slow) may understand something one day but forget it completely later. They may find it difficult to adjust to life in school. Because they learn slowly, they may get bored in class and interrupt the lesson. Often they have other disabilities too. For example, they may find it difficult to make small movements with their fingers such as writing or using scissors.

Some people have **fits**. In other ways, they may be just like other people and should be treated like them. People who have fits are not necessarily mentally handicapped. A person may have a fit only once in his whole life or once a year, once a month or week, or several times a day. In a minor fit, a person may stare without blinking his eyes. In a more serious fit, the person may fall to the ground, make strange cries and shake. Saliva and froth may appear at the mouth. When the fit is over, the person's body relaxes. It can be alarming to see someone with a fit. However, they are not in pain and will not die. It is important to be calm and to reassure others who may be frightened. Ensure that the person is in a safe place where he or she cannot be harmed. Fits cannot spread from one person to another.

Brain damage at birth can cause children to be **spastic** (another name for this is **cerebral palsy**). Their bodies have tight, stiff muscles which they cannot control properly. The legs sometimes cross like scissors.

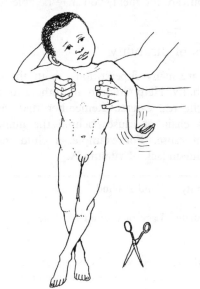

legs crossed like scissors

They may make jerky movements. The face, neck or body may twist. They may or may not be slow mentally. There are no medicines to cure a spastic child. However, they can learn to do many things. Their minds may be quite all right even if they have difficulty in speaking.

Social

In addition to the more obvious problems described above, people may suffer from social disability. Children, in particular, may find that they do not fit in socially at school. Perhaps they have a disability or come from another area and speak a different language. Perhaps they suffer from unhappiness or poverty at home. Perhaps they are thin, fat or pock-marked. For such reasons, they may not be accepted by the other children. This can cause much misery to a child who may become rude and start fights easily; or may become extremely shy and withdrawn. Such a child may be difficult to handle or refuse to go to school. As a teacher, you can sometimes identify the cause of the problem and help the child to become accepted. By showing that you care for them, you may be able to help them.

Causes of disability

There are many superstitions about the causes of disability. Help children and others to understand the real causes. Remember that there is often a chain of causes behind the immediate physical cause. For example, a child may be blind due to lack of vitamin A:

Disability	Child is blind
↑	
Immediate cause	Lack of vitamin A in diet
↑	
Underlying causes	Poverty, food customs and ideas Social, political and economic factors.

In the above table we can see that the immediate cause of the blindness is lack of vitamin A in the diet. But the cause of this is poverty or the kind of food that a child eats. These causes, in turn, depend on social, political and economic factors. You can help people to understand this chain of cause and effect. You can help them to find a way to break the chain and so prevent the disability. You can begin to combat superstitious fear of the unknown through helping to spread knowledge and awareness. **No one should be blamed for a person's disability**.

There are five immediate causes for the majority of disabilities:

Children may be born with the disability

A child may be born deaf, blind or mentally handicapped. Often it is impossible to prevent these disabilities. However, **it is more likely** that a baby will be born healthy if the mother is healthy during pregnancy. Medicines can damage the developing baby, especially during the first three months. Smoking and heavy drinking during pregnancy can also harm a developing baby. The mother should eat well. Her food should contain plenty of energy so she should eat things containing some fats and oils. She also needs protein (see chapter 4). She should eat fruit and dark green vegetables which contains vitamins. She needs iron to prevent anaemia and iodised salt. (Lack of iodine causes certain kinds of brain damage to the baby.) Towards the end of pregnancy she should not do hard physical work.

A baby may become disabled at birth

Some children may be physically or mentally disabled as a result of a difficult birth. Difficult delivery is a common cause of cerebral palsy and fits (see above). The brain may become damaged because it does not get enough oxygen. This can happen if the baby is slow to breathe after birth.

The midwife – the person who helps the mother to deliver the baby – is especially important. She can help to ensure that the baby is born without being damaged. She must see the mother several times during pregnancy. If she thinks that the delivery might be difficult, she should persuade the mother to deliver in hospital. Midwives must know how to make the baby breathe very soon after birth.

Diseases may cause disability

Diseases such as polio, measles, leprosy and whooping cough may cause disability. (See chapter 5 where these diseases are discussed in more detail.) Polio can cause paralysis. Whooping cough can cause fits and death, particularly in young babies. Leprosy causes loss of feeling so that people can burn and injure themselves without realising that they are doing so. Measles can cause blindness, deafness and mental disability. Many of these diseases can be prevented by vaccination and proper health practices. Early treatment is also most important.

Accidents may cause disability

A person may become disabled as a result of an accident at home, at work, or on the roads. (See chapter 6). Children may fall out of trees or burn themselves or injure their eyes. Accidents can happen on the roads. A break in a bone may be badly treated so that the person becomes permanently disabled.

To prevent these accidents, children can learn about these dangers in school. Children and adults can learn simple first aid. Older children can learn how to prevent their younger brothers and sisters from being hurt.

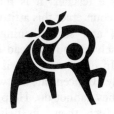

Malnutrition may cause disability

Young children may become disabled if they do not receive enough food or the right kind of food. In severe cases, they may become blind. Sometimes, the brain does not develop properly and the child becomes mentally handicapped. Malnourished children often come from homes that are poor in other ways. They lack mental stimulation and they lack the energy and interest to play. So they do not learn and develop as quickly as well-nourished, mentally stimulated children.

Some Teaching Suggestions

Sometimes it seems that a child's disability is so great that he or she will inevitably lead a dull and dismal life. As a teacher, it is most important that you try to counteract this attitude. By giving children hope, and strengthening their confidence in themselves, you can lead them towards happier lives. In other words, it is important to think **positively**. Concentrate on what they can do, not what they cannot do. Help them to look for ways in which they can help themselves. Encourage other children and adults to understand ways in which they can help the disabled. Spread the idea that disabled people can be helped through **positive action**. In this section, two kinds of positive action for teachers are discussed. First, we suggest practical ideas for coping with disabled children in primary schools. Secondly, we suggest possible ways in which teachers can help normal children to understand the problems of disability.

Disabled children in school

Disabled children may have difficulty in getting to school. Encourage parents, neighbours, other children and other family members to bring these children to school. Ensure that disabled children join in with school activities as far as possible. Below, a girl is taking her blind younger sister to school.

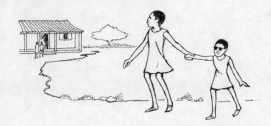

When a disabled child comes to school, talk to the parent or family member who brings him. Try to find out the extent of the disability. What are the child's main difficulties? What can he do? Has he had the disability from birth? Help the parents to understand how the family can help the child with school work. When children first come to school, it is important to try to identify any who may be disabled. It is more difficult to recognise less serious disabilities, for example sight and hearing. Some ideas are given on this in chapter 10.

Teachers have much work to do and many responsibilities. When disabled children are in ordinary schools, this adds to their work and responsibility. If volunteers can be found from the community, they can help to share this load with teachers. They can work with groups of disabled children and give them extra help as necessary during school hours.

Wherever possible, include disabled children in school activities. Many can participate in some sports, scouting, creative activities, regular lessons and school trips. Help them to feel a part of the school. Encourage disabled children to make friends. Both the disabled and the normal children benefit from the relationship. Children can be 'paired' with another child. For example, a sighted child might work with a blind one. Older children can take care of younger ones.

Physically disabled children may not be able to participate in active sports. Remember sometimes to include games where they can join in, such as games which can be played sitting down.

Children often learn better if they work in groups. For the teacher, it needs practice and confidence to let children work like this. Disabled children, however, benefit greatly from working with a group of other children. The other children also benefit. Each learns about the other.

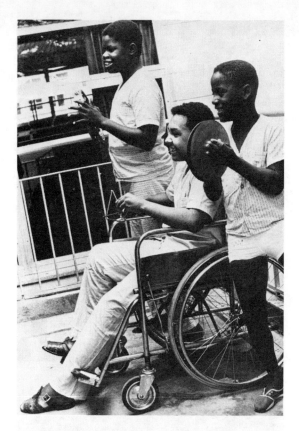

If there are children with hearing difficulties in the class, make sure that they are near the front and can see you. Speak slowly, loudly, and clearly. Remember that your body and face can communicate as much as your voice.

Disabled children often enjoy drawing. Encourage them in this. They may find it easier to use thick crayons or paint.

Children with speech defects can still enjoy drama by miming. Children who cannot move properly may be able to set up a puppet theatre.

Learning and teaching about disability

It is important that normal children should learn about the problems of the disabled and how they can help.

Explain about disability. Talk with the class about it. Read the background information above. Here are some questions to start children talking:

- Do you know a child who cannot run or walk like you?
- Why can't the child run or walk like you?
- Why do some children not play with this child?
- Can the child play some of your games?
- Do other children laugh at this child?
- What is it like when other children laugh at you?
- Would you like to be disabled?
- Do you like having friends?
- How would you feel if you were disabled and had no friends?
- Do you like playing with other children?
- What can disabled people do better than you can do?
- How can you help disabled people to enjoy better lives?

Discuss the causes of disability and emphasise that no one is to blame for it.

All children, including the disabled, enjoy music. Even deaf children can feel the vibrations from the music. Mentally handicapped children often enjoy the rhythm of music. Encourage all children to participate.

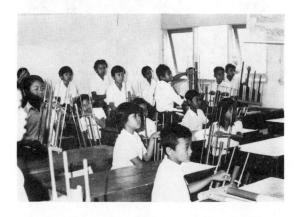

Play a game. A game or role play can help your children to understand more about disabled children.

One child pretends to have a disability. For example, he might pretend to have a stiff leg so that he cannot walk properly. Make the disability as realistic as possible. Tie a stick to one or both legs. It is difficult for the child to run. He cannot bend his leg. Now the children play a running game like football or tag. After a few minutes, let another child be the one with the disability. All the children can play the game. They behave in different ways towards the child with the limp. Some help him. Some laugh at him. Some are friendly. Some do not talk to him. Let the children think of ways to behave.

Let children play games about other disabilities such as blind or deaf children. Then talk about what happened.

Ask the children questions:

- What was it like being handicapped?
- What did you feel?
- Did you like it? Why not?
- What did the other children feel?

Remember that children usually behave well to a child with a very bad disability. They are often more cruel to a child with a small disability.

Tell a story. Here is a story called 'Koffi and the Magic Stick'. Read this story and think about how you would use it with a class of children. What points would you try to bring out from the story? Children could make drawings to illustrate parts of the story. Could they act a short play based on it?

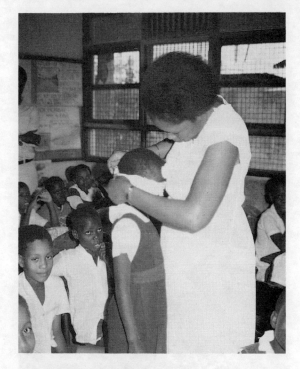

'Being blind': a role play

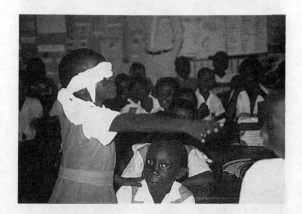

Koffi and the Magic Stick

Koffi is a small boy who lives in a small village in Africa. Koffi was not able to see from the time he was born. He was a blind child. So Koffi could not see that the sky is blue and the grass is green.

When he was a baby, his mother let him crawl around while she did her housework. Koffi tried to use his hands to feel all the things in the house.

When it was time to eat, Koffi would know where to find his plate and mug which his mother always left in the same place for Koffi. At first, his mother would feed him because she liked to do this. But Koffi did not like that very much and soon learned to eat by himself with his fingers.

When mother took the clothes down to the lake to wash, she took Koffi with her. He loved going down to the lake because mother would let him stand in the water and bathe himself. He loved to feel the water on his face and to splash about with his hands and feet.

Because it was so quiet by the lake, Koffi could hear the birds singing in the trees. He learned to know the song and chatter of the different birds.

One day after washing the clothes, Mother and Koffi were walking back through the jungle path. Koffi could feel the wind blowing in the trees and was afraid, so he held Mother's hand. Mother knew that a big storm was coming so she told Koffi not to be afraid. Koffi could not see that suddenly it got dark because of the storm, but he felt that the air was cooler and soon felt the raindrops on his face. So Mother picked Koffi up in her arms and hurried home. Neither she nor Koffi got wet.

When Koffi was a little bigger and could run around by himself, his brothers and sisters took him to the village market on Saturdays. Koffi loved to hear the voices of the people selling their wares. One day he was listening so hard to all the voices around him that he was not careful about where he was walking. Suddenly Koffi's foot caught on a stone and he fell down. While he was trying to stand up, Koffi's hand touched a stick. He used this stick to help him stand up. From that time on, Koffi and the stick became very good friends. He had a name for the stick because it was his best friend. The name was Magic.

Koffi took Magic with him wherever he went, holding it in his hand and moving it in front of him. Magic became Koffi's eyes. It would tell him if there were rocks and trees on the path so that Koffi could be careful where he walked. Now he seldom fell down.

Soon Koffi was six years old. It was time for him to go to school. Magic went to school with him, showing him the way. On the first day, Koffi was afraid to go to school alone so Koffi's big brother went with him and took him to the teacher.

Teacher introduced Koffi to all the other children in the class and told them that they must help Koffi because he could not see. Koffi liked his teacher.

When it was time to learn to write his name, Teacher gave Koffi a tray with sand on it. Teacher showed him how to write in the sand with his finger. Soon Koffi could write his own name. He also learned to write the name of Marie who sat beside him in the class. Koffi used his tray of sand not only to write his name but also to do the sums that Teacher had taught him.

Every day, before it was time to go home, Teacher read a story to the class from a book. Koffi liked to listen to the stories but he could not read. His friend, Marie, would read a story to him after they had played together in the evening. Marie also helped Koffi to do his lessons.

Koffi learned many things in school and looked forward to going to school every day. During the holidays, Koffi liked to go for long walks. Sometimes he went with Marie and his school friends, and sometimes he went alone with Magic. Wherever he went, Koffi always took Magic with him.

When Koffi had finished his studies at the village school, he went to live in the big city far away and learned to be a teacher. Marie too learned to be a teacher.

Now Koffi and Marie are married and back in their village. The village now has many more people, so the school is much bigger. Koffi and Marie are both teachers in the school that they went to together as little children.

There are many important points in this story. Read the section on Story Telling in Chapter 8. Pick out the points of the story to which you would draw the children's attention.

Children can begin to understand the problems of deaf children if they try to communicate without speaking. Can they make up a **sign language?** Can they make a sign language which everyone in the school and community can use? In the figure below are some suggestions. However, let children work out signs for themselves. They don't have to use the ones shown here. They could try to communicate messages using their sign language rather than sound.

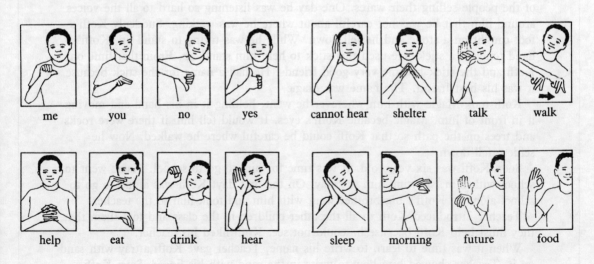

| me | you | no | yes | cannot hear | shelter | talk | walk |

| help | eat | drink | hear | sleep | morning | future | food |

Make some aids. Older children could help to make some aids for physically disabled children. Here are some ideas for a back rest, floor seat, walking bars and climbing frame.

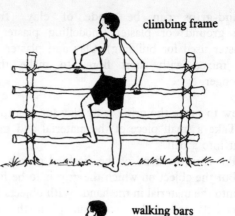

climbing frame

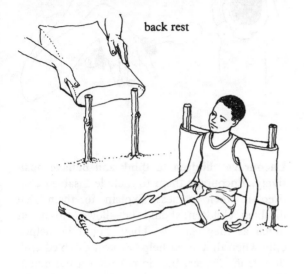

back rest

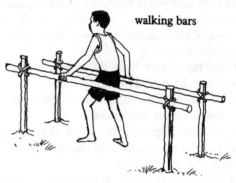

walking bars

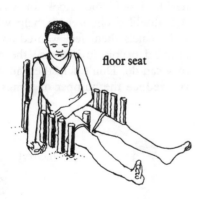

floor seat

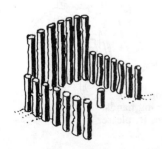

Another useful aid which older children could make is a hand-grip. Hand-grips can help a person whose hand is disabled to hold many things. Here are some of the types of hand disability which people may have:

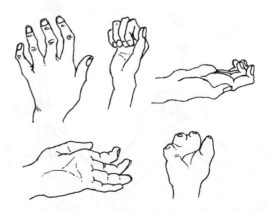

Hand-grips can be made of clay (from the ground) or plaster (modelling plaster or plaster used for building). Clay and plaster can be mixed with short fibres to make them stronger.

How to make the grip (using clay for example)

1 Take a small piece of the material and make it into a ball.
2 Put it in the hand of the disabled person.
3 Put the object on which the grip is to be fixed into the material in the hand. With objects like pencils and forks, you can push the end through the material. Do not wrap the clay around the pencil.
4 Make the person hold the object in the way in which he would normally use it.
5 Press the person's fingers firmly into position to make a clear impression.
6 Leave the grip in place for a few minutes. Then take the object with the grip out of the hand and let it harden.
7 If the grip is made of clay, bake it in the sun. Cover with oil or grease to make it more resistant to water. Do not immerse the grip in water if you are washing the object.

Here are some things which can be held in a hand-grip by a disabled person:

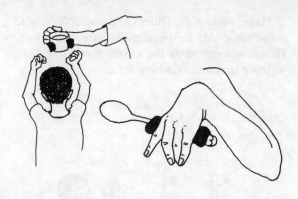

Encourage children to think and behave positively. Encourage them to include disabled children in their games. Explain to them that disabled children should be allowed to do as much as they can do. They should be helped only when they need help. Protect disabled children from danger, but do not protect too much! Too much protection can be dangerous for the health of any child. Look for what they **can** do. Ask disabled children to help where they can. This makes them feel wanted and useful. Help disabled people to **increase** the range of things they can do. Don't help them in such a way that you **reduce** the number of things that they do.

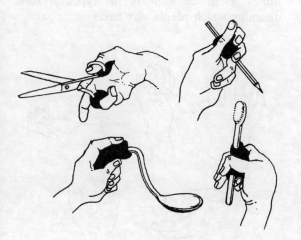

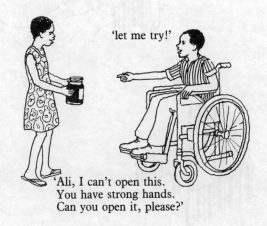

'let me try!'

'Ali, I can't open this. You have strong hands. Can you open it, please?'

Useful Background Knowledge

The other sex

Many children in the higher forms of the primary school have entered puberty. (Puberty means the time when a child becomes sexually mature.) It is a time when young people experience strong sexual feelings. Often, they do not quite understand how to cope with these feelings. They realise that they will soon be adults but they know that, in many ways, they are still children. 'Sex' represents an exciting but perhaps worrying new world for them.

You may not feel able to handle this difficult and sensitive subject. Only you can judge the situation.

You must take into account:

- The religious and moral ideas of the society in which you live.
- The views of the community in which you live. Maybe parents think that teachers should have nothing to do with sex education.
- Your own sense of confidence. Does it embarrass you to talk about sex?
- Are you worried by children's questions?
- Your relationship with the children. It is essential that they like and trust you and know that you are trying to help them. If you can create a firm, gentle, friendly, good-humoured, sympathetic atmosphere in your class, children will feel able to discuss their problems. Sex education is impossible in an ill-disciplined, noisy class which has no sense of direction.

You may decide that this is not a subject which you want to tackle. On the other hand, you may want to be prepared to answer children's questions if they raise them. If so, you may find that the following background information is useful. It is given in some detail so that at least **you** know the 'facts'. Remember that many adolescents obtain information about sex from each other. They often find it easier to talk to their friends than to adults. The problem is that the information which they obtain may not be accurate. Sometimes this wrong information can make children very worried or unhappy. Remember, too, that language is very important. Children should know the proper words which we use to describe our sex or genital organs and their functions.

How the body changes

Both boys and girls need to know about the changes which take place in their bodies at the time of puberty. The diagrams shown here summarise these changes. Girls usually enter puberty before boys. They are often more physically mature than boys of the same age. Children's development at this time happens differently. Each has his or her own time-scale. The progress of development is controlled by a tiny gland in the brain. The gland is called the **pituitary**. It produces hormones (chemical substances) which enter the blood and which make the sex organs develop. The sex organs, in turn, produce hormones which control the changes in the other parts of the bodies of boys and girls.

Adolescence can often be a difficult time. As well as these physical changes, there are mental and emotional changes. Children are becoming adults. They begin to resent authority. They experience strong sexual and emotional feelings. They are becoming more independent but do not yet have full adult responsibility. Teachers can help and reassure them. Adolescents need sympathy and firmness, tactful advice and understanding.

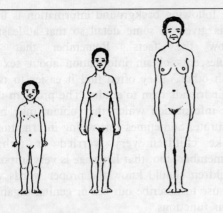

How girls will change:
gradual development of breasts
rounding of hips
growth of hair under arms and around vagina
sweat glands become more active
start of menstruation (periods)
attraction to opposite sex

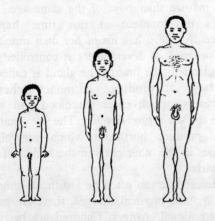

How boys will change:
growth of hair under arms, on chest, face, and around penis
penis and testicles grow bigger
voice begins to change
testicles begin to produce sperm
sweat glands become more active
attraction to opposite sex

How babies are made

A woman's sex organs inside her body look like this:

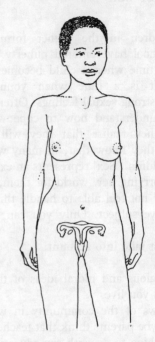

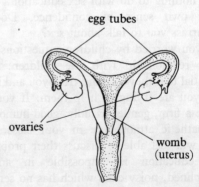

egg tubes

ovaries

womb (uterus)

Remember that there are other organs inside her abdomen as well! This is a simplified diagram to show only the sex organs.

The ovaries of the woman contain eggs (or **ova**, singular **ovum**). The eggs are very tiny, no bigger than the full stop at the end of this sentence. From the time of puberty the ovaries release one egg about every twenty eight days. This egg can pass down the Fallopian tube (or egg tube) to the uterus. If it is fertilised by a sperm from a man, it will develop into a baby.

At the time of puberty, many changes take place in the body of a girl. They begin to **menstruate**. Their bodies go through a cycle (the **menstrual cycle**) lasting about twenty eight days. After an egg is released from the ovary, the lining of the uterus becomes thicker. The uterus is where the egg will grow and develop if it is fertilised. If this happened, the lining would provide the oxygen and food for the egg's development. Usually, however, the egg is not fertilised, so the lining is not required. It falls off and pases out through the vagina, causing bleeding. This bleeding is called **menstruation** or a **monthly period**. A girl can wear a pad to catch this blood. Sometimes, she may wear a special pad inside her vagina called a **tampon**. The pad protects her clothes and makes her feel more comfortable. The monthly period lasts for about 3 to 5 days. It is a perfectly natural event but can be worrying to young girls. Teachers and parents can reassure girls that it is a normal part of growing up.

At about 45–50, a woman stops producing eggs and her periods stop. This time is called the **menopause**.

In boys also, a number of changes happen to their bodies at the time of puberty. Sperms begin to be made in two small oval balls (**testes**) which hang in a bag of skin (the **scrotum**) behind the penis.

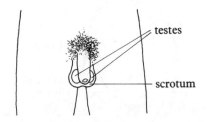

The ovaries in a girl produce only one egg at a time. But the testes in a boy make millions of sperms. Sperms are much smaller than eggs. You can see them only through a microscope. They look like this:

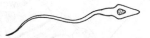

The sperms are stored in the testes in tiny tubes. Certain glands produce a sticky liquid in which the sperms pass through the penis. If the body is viewed in section, it would look like this:

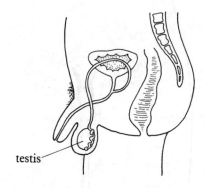

So many sperm cells are produced by the testes that they sometimes spill out through the penis. This can happen when the body is relaxed during sleep. It is often accompanied by a vivid dream and is therefore called a 'wet dream'. It is a perfectly natural occurrence.

Sexual intercourse and fertilisation

When a man and a woman make love, they feel tender towards each other. The man's penis becomes hard and this is called **erection**. When the penis is hard, he can put it into the woman's vagina.

After a time, semen comes out. The semen contains several million sperms which swim through the vagina, into the uterus and up the Fallopian tube.

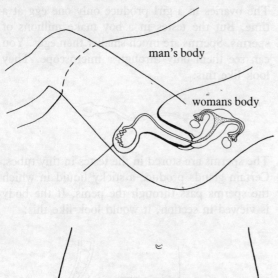

man's body

womans body

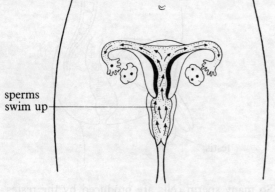

sperms swim up

If the sperms meet an egg in this tube, one of them may fertilise it. The sperm goes into the egg and becomes part of it. The moment when the sperm and egg join is called fertilisation. After the egg is fertilised, it divides into two, then into four and so on until it forms a solid ball of cells. This ball of cells passes down the fallopian tube and into the uterus. It buries or embeds itself in the thickened lining of the uterus. It divides into two parts. One part becomes the **placenta** which stays attached to the wall of the uterus. The other part develops into the baby, which floats in a bag of fluid. The lining of the uterus is needed now, so menstruation stops.

The development of the baby and birth

The part of the egg which develops into the baby is called the **embryo**. By twelve weeks, this embryo is more or less complete. Then it is called a **foetus**. It has limbs, organs such as heart and lungs and a brain.

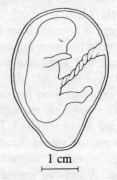

1 cm

Because development happens so fast during these first twelve weeks, this is a very important time. During this time, the embryo can easily be injured. (This can occur, for example, if the mother gets a disease called German Measles, if she smokes a lot, or takes drugs.)

The foetus is living. It needs food and oxygen. This is supplied from the mother through the placenta. The blood systems of the baby and mother are separate but close to each other. Thus, food and oxygen can pass from the blood of the mother to the baby. Carbon dioxide and other wastes can pass from the baby's blood to the mother's. This exchange takes place in the placenta.

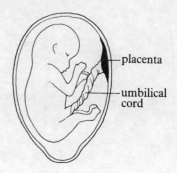

placenta

umbilical cord

The tube which connects the placenta to the baby is called the umbilical cord. It carries the food, oxygen and waste products between placenta and baby. When the baby is ready to be born, the umbilical cord is about 50 cm long.

From about twenty weeks, the baby is fairly active inside the mother. She can feel the movements which the baby makes. The baby is contained inside a watery liquid which helps to protect it.

After about nine months from the time of fertilisation, the baby is ready to be born.

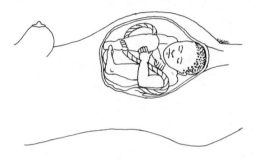

The mother goes into a period of 'labour'. The strong muscle of the uterus begins to contract automatically. (The uterus works hard which is why it is called 'labour'.) Normally the head, which is the biggest part of the baby, comes out first.

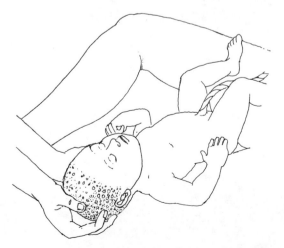

The baby passes to the outside world through the vagina which is elastic and can stretch. The umbilical cord is tied or clamped in two places. It is cut between the two clamps. The baby cries and begins to breathe air through its lungs. The piece of umbilical cord attached to the baby drops off some days later leaving a scar – the navel. Soon the placenta comes away from the walls of the uterus and is passed out through the mother's vagina.

The baby's sex

A baby's sex is determined by the **sperms**. Two kinds of sperm are made in the testes. One kind will produce a boy baby and one kind will produce a girl baby. Slightly more 'male' sperms are produced than 'female' sperms.

Twins

Sometimes two eggs, which are fertilised by two different sperms, are released from the ovaries. They develop into two separate babies which may be of either sex. They are called **non-identical** twins. Sometimes, however, early in its development one fertilised egg divides into two. The two twins are said to be **identical** because they develop from one egg and one sperm. They must, of course, be of the same sex. Identical twins are very unusual.

Contraception

It is possible to prevent fertilisation – and therefore the birth of a baby – by various methods. For example, fertilisation of an egg is likely to take place only at certain times in a woman's menstrual cycle. There is a time in the cycle, a few days before and after the menstrual period, when fertilisation is unlikely (the **safe** period). This method is not very reliable because it is difficult to know exactly when an egg is released. Another method of contraception is the **pill**. By taking a pill every day, the woman prevents eggs from being released by the ovaries. If she takes these pills correctly, it is unlikely that she will become pregnant. She can have injections every three months which work the same way as the pill. Other methods of contraception physically prevent the egg and sperm from meeting. For example, a woman can wear a **cap** inside her vagina. A man can wear a **condom** over his penis during intercourse. These methods are not quite so reliable as the pill. Another important method of contraception is 'the **loop**' or 'coil'. This is a small plastic or copper coil which is put into the uterus. It prevents the fertilised egg from embedding in the wall of the uterus. It should be put in by a doctor or health worker.

Remember that the subject of contraception may be controversial in the society in which you live. Some religions approve only of certain methods.

Some Teaching Suggestions

Teaching about sex is difficult. People often have strong views about whether the subject should be discussed, particularly in school. Children may feel embarrassed. You, as the teacher, may also feel embarrassed or uncomfortable. Religious and cultural beliefs, social customs and individual attitudes are all involved.

The biological 'facts' explained above are only a small part of sex, for sex affects many aspects of our lives. It concerns our relationships with other people. It concerns our deepest feelings. It concerns the making and development of babies, new human beings. It concerns our physical and emotional well-being. It can give us great pleasure – and great pain.

Only you can judge, for your situation and circumstances, how to handle this subject. What does the official curriculum say? What are the customs of the local community? In many countries, especially in Africa and Asia, children grow up in very crowded homes. They learn the facts of life, about sex and babies, very early. Often, they have to look after a younger baby brother or sister.

In your training course to become a teacher, you might like to discuss this issue. Should teachers regard sex and reproduction as part of health education for young children? After all, these days we say we are encouraging children to have enquiring minds. Should we therefore be surprised if they ask us questions about their own origins?

Here are some important points to remember:

- You cannot answer children's questions properly if you feel embarrassed and shy. Often children simply want straightforward information at a level they can understand. Suppose a child of six asks: 'Did I come out of my Mummy's tummy?' He may well just be seeking assurance, to confirm what he already half knows. He doesn't want or expect a half hour lecture on sexual intercourse. So, as a teacher, you have to try to determine what kind of information children are seeking and adjust your answers accordingly.

- Children often use or invent their own words to describe their sex organs. Or they may use common slang. If proper words exist in your own language, you should use them. If you are teaching in English you should teach children the proper English words (sperm, vagina, penis, umbilical cord etc.).

- When you discuss a subject like this with children, you need the right atmosphere in the classroom. You need to know the children well. You need to know the kinds of homes which they come from. Are their parents farmers or workers in a city? Are they Moslem or Christian? Are they of another religion? Is the subject ever discussed in their homes? Try not to be shocked by the children's ideas. Listen to them and accept what they say. Never mock or laugh at their ideas.

- Remember that children copy adults. They usually copy what we **do** rather than what we **say**. They learn their maleness or femaleness from the adults around them, especially their parents, but also from their teachers. Whether consciously or unconsciously, children learn from adults how men and women behave. Parents and teachers have a great responsibility.

With younger children

The following ideas are the most important:

- living things come from living things
- like comes from like
- human babies (and other mammals) grow inside their mothers before they are born
- you need both a man and a woman to make a baby

How and when you teach about this will depend on the opportunities which arise. For example, if one of the children has had a recent baby brother or sister, you could use this as a starting point. You could discuss where the baby came from. You could discuss where the children think **they** came from.

Other activities might include:

● Hatching out toad's eggs in a simple polythene bag aquarium or looking at baby chicks.
● You could ask who has seen a goat or calf or rabbit being born. Get the children to describe this and to talk about it.
● You, or you and the children together, could make a big chart to put on the classroom wall.

An example is shown at the bottom of the page.

You could use simple flash cards together with the chart. For example:

| kitten | calf | baby |

● Use pictures from magazines and newspapers. Put them on a wall of your classroom. Use pictures done by the children. Can children make drawings of young animals? Can they match these to the adults? Do they understand that a goat always produces a goat – and never a dog or a cat, or a donkey?

Try this: you are teaching the first-year children in a primary school. You have been teaching them for a term. You know the children well. A child asks you how babies are made. All the children are quiet and listen. What will you say?

With older children

Older children may want to know some of the information given above under the heading 'Useful Background Knowledge'. Open discussion is one approach which may be suitable. However, remember that children and young people may be embarrassed to ask questions openly. They may be afraid to show their ignorance in front of the class. Or they may be worried about something that they have heard or seen. One solution is to ask the children to write their questions down. Tell them not to write their names on the paper. Let them put the questions in a box. You can then read them later and answer them in a discussion session. Do not be shocked by the questions. They are probably not being cheeky! They want to know about something which concerns them deeply. As teachers, we have to learn how to respond to their doubts, needs and uncertainties – sensitively and skilfully. As older and more mature people, we can help to shape children's attitudes towards, and understanding of, one of the fundamental aspects of human existence.

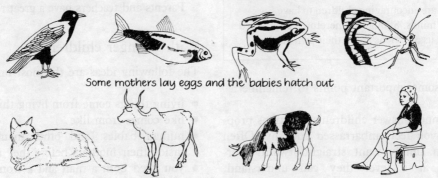

Some mothers lay eggs and the babies hatch out

Many mothers have babies which are born alive

66

Chapter Four

Food and health

Useful Background Knowledge

The children below are well nourished.

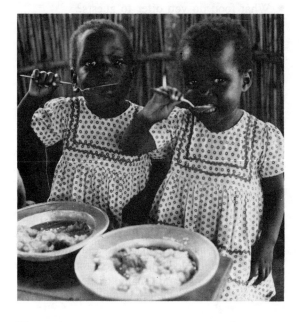

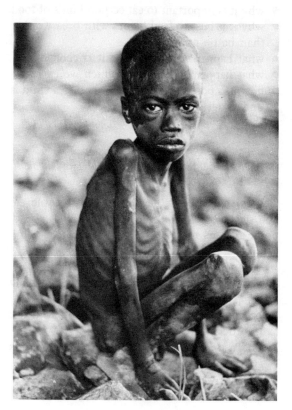

If people do not eat anything, they die. If they do not eat enough they become sick and thin. The child in the photo above right has not had enough food. We say that he is undernourished. Throughout the world, one out of every three children is undernourished.

In some countries, two out of every three children are undernourished. If children are undernourished, their mental and physical growth and development are handicapped. Thus, knowledge

In the whole world

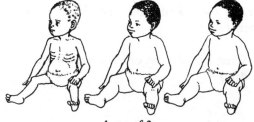

1 out of 3

about food and nutrition is important. It is knowledge which can save life and directly affects the health and happiness of people.

As a teacher, you can help to spread knowledge about food and nutrition. You can help children – and through children their families – to understand:

- why it is important to eat certain kinds of food
- why it is best to feed babies with breast rather than bottle milk
- what happens to food when it is cooked
- what happens to the food which we eat
- how it is possible to find out whether a child is undernourished

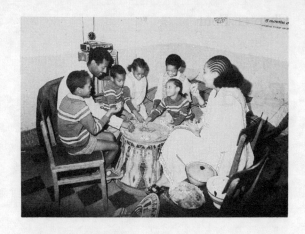

Why do we eat and drink?

Let us think about the reasons why people eat and drink

Some reasons may be the five 'H's':

- because our stomachs feel empty (**Hunger**)
- because it is the time of day when we normally eat (**Habit**)
- because we know that we need food and drink in order to live (**Health**)
- because we enjoy eating certain foods (**Happiness**)
- because we have guests and it is a custom to offer them food and drink (**Hospitality**)

There are many customs associated with eating and drinking. Some people use chopsticks. Some people use a knife and fork. Some people use their fingers.

- What food do you eat at home? What do you drink?

- What food do you offer to guests?
- What food and drink are not allowed according to your custom?
- What food and drink do you have on special occasions, (weddings, for example)?

Many eating and drinking habits are social or religious. Sometimes we do not eat or drink certain foods or we fast because of religious taboos, or social custom. Often we eat particular foods because they are cheap and easily available.

But sometimes people waste money and risk their health on expensive foods and drinks which are not good for them. These include 'junk' foods such as pre-packaged snacks, sweets and drinks. They are high in sugar and low in real nutrient value. Alcoholic drinks, too, result in family problems and malnourished children. They can cause drunkenness and misery.

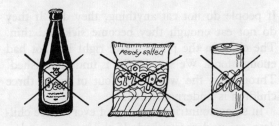

Foods for health

What do **you** eat and drink every day?
What food and drink do you have:

- at the beginning of the day
- during the day
- in the evening
- when guests come to your home
- when you go out with your friends

Keep a diary for a week, to show what you eat and drink. (This is also something you can do with children in primary school.)
You could arrange your diary like this:

	Morning	Daytime	Evening
Monday			
Tuesday			
Wednesday			
Thursday			
Friday			
Saturday			
Sunday			

Make sure that you leave enough space in each column to write what you eat and drink. Collect together the results from your fellow students. Make a bar chart like this:

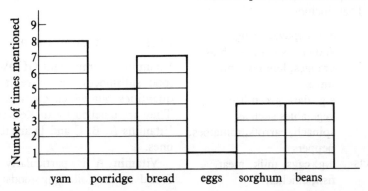

Which foods are mentioned most often? Why do you think they are so popular? Do you think these are the most popular foods everywhere in the world? Discuss the results of this exercise among yourselves and with your tutor. You will probably find that there are one or two **main** foods in your diet. Depending on where you live, these may be:
Cereals and grains, for example, rice, sorghum, wheat, maize, millet.
Starchy roots, for example, yam, cassava, potato.
Starchy fruits, for example, breadfruit, banana.
These are very important. They are cheap, plentiful and are often the main item in people's diets.
Foods contain several kinds of NUTRIENT:

Carbohydrates Fats and Oils	These provide energy for the body
Protein	This is necessary for the healthy growth of the body including bones, muscles and the brain
Vitamins Minerals	They help the body to work properly and keep it healthy. Minerals are necessary for healthy blood, bones and teeth

The main food which people eat is called the **staple** food. It contains **carbohydrate**. Some staple foods, such as cereals, also contain protein. Other staple foods such as root crops like yam or cassava contain little protein. Some staple foods contain vitamins.

To eat a healthy and well balanced diet, we have to add foods which are rich in the other nutrients. We can call these 'helper' foods the GO – GROW – GLOW foods.

The GO helper foods contain energy in a more concentrated form than the staple foods. Fats, for example, contain two or three times as much energy for the same weight as the staple food. Examples of GO foods are:

- Fats and oils   e.g. cooking oil, butter, 'ghee', groundnuts, milk, avocado, fatty meat, coconut
- Sugars   e.g. sugar, sugar cane, honey, molasses

The GROW helper foods are rich in protein. The staple food may contain some protein but the GROW helper foods have more protein of a higher quality. Examples of GROW foods are:

- Animal products   e.g. chicken, meat, milk, eggs, fish
- Legumes   e.g. peas, soya beans, groundnuts
- Nuts and certain seeds   e.g. walnuts, cashew nuts, sunflower seeds

The GLOW helper foods are rich in minerals and vitamins. The importance of them is further explained below. They include:

- Fruits   e.g. papaya, mango, and citrus fruits such as oranges, lemons, and limes
- Vegetables   e.g. dark green leafy vegetables such as spinach, carrots, tomatoes, peppers
- Animal products   e.g. eggs, milk, meat, fish, chicken

You will see from this that many foods are rich in more than one nutrient. Groundnuts, for example, are good GROW and GO helpers. This diagram summarises the above ideas:

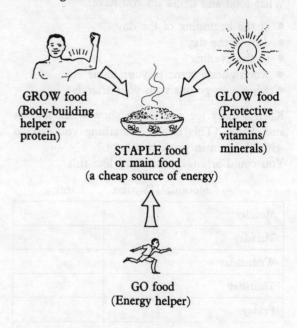

GROW food (Body-building helper or protein)

GLOW food (Protective helper or vitamins/minerals)

STAPLE food or main food (a cheap source of energy)

GO food (Energy helper)

Look again at your food diary. What was the STAPLE food? What were the GO, GROW, and GLOW foods in each meal? Make a meal plan for every day in one week. Work out how much each meal costs. See how cheaply you can make a meal which includes food from each group.

More about vitamins and minerals

Vitamins are important GLOW foods. They are food substances which we need in very small quantities but which are vital for good health. They are labelled by the letters of the alphabet. Vitamins A, B, C and D are the most important ones.

Vitamin A is particularly important. It is found in the following foods: dark green leafy vegetables; fruits and vegetables coloured red and yellow (carrots and papaya and red palm oil for example). In some places, people suffer from a lack of it. If this continues for a long time, they become blind. The vitamin is needed for the sensitive cells of the eye upon which light falls (the retina). An early sign or symptom of vitamin A deficiency is night blindness. That is the person cannot see well in the dark. Later the eye becomes dry, and changes so much that the person becomes blind.

Vitamin B includes several different vitamins. These are found in cereals, especially the brown cereals. White rice and plain flour contain less vitamins so they are not so healthy.

Vitamin C is found in oranges, lemons, guavas and green vegetables. Lack of vitamin C causes a range of symptoms and diseases. Wounds are slow to heal and scar tissue does not form properly. Bleeding from the mouth and gums occurs. If people eat plenty of fruit and green vegetables, lack of vitamin C is unlikely to be a problem.

Vitamin D is made in people's skin through the action of sunlight. We also get this vitamin from milk. It is necessary for the proper formation of bones. People may lack vitamin D if they live in communities where they have to stay indoors. They may also lack it if they have to cover their skin with clothes so that the sun does not reach the skin. This can occur with women in some Moslem communities.

Certain minerals are also important GLOW foods. **Iron** and **Iodine** are two minerals which people sometimes lack. Iron is necessary to form the red part of the blood. If people do not have enough, they suffer from anaemia. Beans, green vegetables and certain fruits such as figs are rich in iron. Iodine is used by the thyroid gland which is in the neck. If the thyroid gland does not get enough iodine, it swells up giving a lump in the neck region. In many places, iodine is now added to the salt which is sold in shops and markets.

> **Remember**
> For a well balanced diet, we should try to eat GO, GROW, GLOW foods **in addition** to the STAPLE food. The STAPLE food is very important. It usually provides, in addition to energy, half or more of the body's needed vitamins and proteins.

Food for children

Young children need food (in addition to breast milk) from the age of 4–6 months. They **do not** need food, other than breast milk, before this. It is especially important to add the GO – GROW – GLOW foods to a young child's food. The STAPLE food alone is not enough because STAPLE foods are bulky (this means large in volume for the energy value which they contain). They also contain a lot of water. A child's stomach is small and he cannot eat enough STAPLE food to give him all the nutrients which he needs. The GO – GROW – GLOW foods can provide the extra nutrients without making the volume of food larger. So the child gets **more** nourishment from a **smaller** meal.

If children lack food, they will not grow. If they eat only the STAPLE food, they will become ill. The child below does not eat enough. He has dry malnutrition or marasmus. He is just skin and bones.

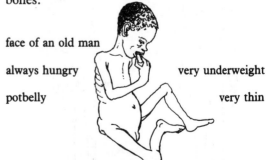

face of an old man

always hungry   very underweight

potbelly   very thin

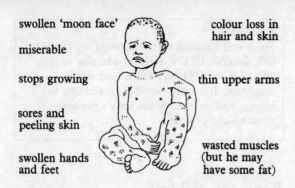

swollen 'moon face'

miserable

stops growing

sores and
peeling skin

swollen hands
and feet

colour loss in
hair and skin

thin upper arms

wasted muscles
(but he may
have some fat)

For every seriously malnourished child, there are many more who are under-weight and not growing well. The child above has a lot to eat but they are all energy foods. He does not get enough GROW and GLOW foods. He has wet malnutrition or kwashiorkor. He is just skin, bones and water.

How to find under-weight children (if you cannot actually weigh them)

The thickness of a young child's upper arm is usually a good indicator of whether he is well nourished (properly fed) or not. This is true when the child is between one and five years old.

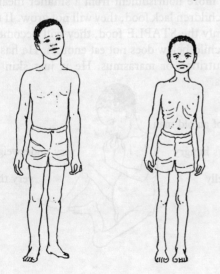

If a child is well-nourished he has fairly thick arms and legs.

If he is poorly-nourished he has very thin arms and legs

Which one of these children in the picture below left is well-nourished?

Measuring a child's upper arm:

This can be done in several ways. You can use a small bracelet and see if it fits onto the child's arm.

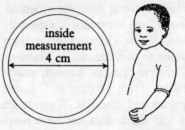

inside
measurement
4 cm

If the bracelet
will not slide
past the elbow,
the child is
well nourished

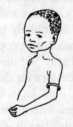

If the bracelet
slides easily
onto the upper
arm, the child is
poorly nourished

Or you could cut a thin strip about 25 cm in length from a material which does not stretch. This could be X-ray film, heavy cloth, or thick paper. Mark along it the measurements as shown on page 73. Colour the areas as shown. Put the strip around the upper arm of children between one and five years old. You can practise using the strip on older children (where it will not be correct), and on other things such as bamboo canes, cans, or bottles.

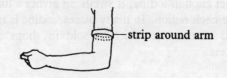

strip around arm

Food for babies

From birth to four months

Breast milk is the best complete food for babies up to 4–6 months old. In fact, breast milk alone is enough up to the age of 4–6 months.

> REMEMBER: BREAST IS BEST

If a mother thinks that she does not have enough milk, she can increase her milk by:

- making sure that the baby has the nipple and the dark skin around it well into his mouth
- feeding the baby very often for a few days and every time that he cries
- resting more, and drinking extra fluid for a few days

She should not give other food or milk, since they take away the baby's appetite. The baby will not suck at the breast, and this **causes** the mother's milk to dry up.

Why breast milk is best:

From 4–6 months to a year

The child can now have other foods as well as breast milk. These foods need to be cooked well and mashed until soft. Start with a simple gruel made from the STAPLE food. After a week or two, begin to add a little of the GO, GROW, GLOW foods. If some oil or fat is added, this helps to make the food soft for the baby as well as adding energy. At first, babies need only a little food once or twice a day until they are used to eating. Breast milk is still the main food. By the age of nine months, they need to eat at least three times a day. By the age of one year, they need a meal or snack about five times a day. The child's stomach is still small. If he eats more often, he is more likely to get enough food.

Food for mothers

When women are pregnant they need to eat more food than before – especially the GO, GROW and GLOW foods. They need extra iron and

For the child	For the mother
1 It contains exactly what the baby needs	1 It is very cheap
2 It contains no germs	2 It does not have to be prepared
3 Feeding helps the baby and mother to love each other	3 It helps mothers to lose weight again after the baby is born
4 Substances in the milk help to protect the baby against diarrhoea and other infections	
5 Babies who do not feed at the breast often get sick and grow very slowly	

73

vitamins to keep their blood strong enough. Mothers who do not eat enough give birth to smaller, weaker babies.

There may be some customs in your area which stop pregnant women from eating some healthy foods. Make a list of those foods which are forbidden. Are any of them foods which women **should** eat to be healthy and to produce healthy babies?

We need to overcome this conflict between custom and good health. Look at your list of forbidden foods. Do these conflict with foods a mother **should** eat?

A mother who has just had a baby also needs to eat more food than before, especially the GO, GROW, GLOW foods. Do mothers in your area eat well? If not, what are the reasons?

Cooking and storing food

If you cook food in too much water, or for too long, or with soda, you can lose many of the vitamins. Baking and steaming food helps to keep the vitamins in.

If food is kept over from one meal to another it should be tightly covered to keep out flies and other insects which carry infection. Try to keep out ants too. Put the covered food on a table and stand the legs of the table in tins or dishes of water.

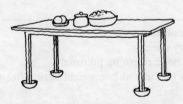

Fly wire or other fine mesh wire can be useful when covering food. Flies and other insects can carry germs to food, thus spreading disease. (See chapter 5).

Food should be kept as cool as possible. Refrigerators are often too expensive, so it is important to find the coolest place in the house. Food should never be kept so long that it smells. Usually it is a good idea to cook only as much food as you need for each meal. Dried or baked foods, such as bread or biscuits, will keep for a few days in an airtight tin.

If food needs to be kept (particularly meat or fish) you can keep it in salt. But before eating it, be sure to rinse a lot of boiled water through it and soak it in water which is free of salt. This will get rid of the salt. Salt is good for us if we sweat a lot in hot weather (it will stop cramp) but too much salt will make us thirsty and is bad for blood pressure. Another way of keeping meat or fish for a short time is to smoke it.

Dried maize (corn), if soaked in lime before cooking, is richer in calcium, and allows more of the vitamins and protein to be used by the body. Rice and other grains are better in health value if their inner skins are left on. Whole rice and wheat contain more vitamins than the white product.

Always make sure cooking and storing pots are clean and are washed after every meal.

What happens to food?

What happens to food when it is eaten? Where does it go? What changes happen? How does the food which we eat change into our bodies?

There are two important processes to understand. These are **digestion** and **absorption**. First, food has to be **digested**. This means that the nutrients must be broken down chemically into simpler substances. They can then be **absorbed** into the bloodstream and carried around the body.

Digestion takes place in the long 'tube' which runs from the mouth to the anus.

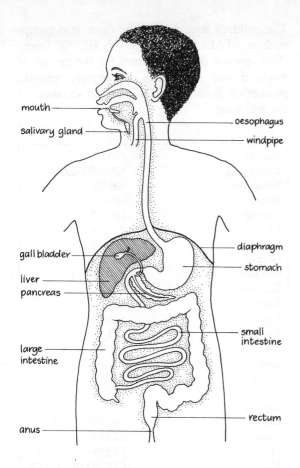

mouth
salivary gland
oesophagus
windpipe
gall bladder
diaphragm
stomach
liver
pancreas
large intestine
small intestine
rectum
anus

It can contract and churn the food, mixing it thoroughly. Glands in the stomach produce an acid which can kill most of the germs on the food.

From the stomach the mixed food passes into the **small intestine**. It is here that absorption takes place. The small intestine is a coiled tube about six metres long. Here, bile from the liver, and juices from the pancreas and small intestine itself are added to the food. The juices contain special chemicals called **enzymes** which can break down the nutrients into simpler food substances. The food is now in the form of a thin liquid which can be absorbed into the bloodstream. The food substances which the body needs pass through the walls of the small intestine into the blood. Once the food is in the blood, it can be taken all around the body.

The food which is not absorbed passes into the **large intestine**. This is shorter but wider than the small intestine. Water is absorbed into the blood here. The remaining waste products are stored here. Later, they are pushed out of the body as faeces (a 'stool'). Much of this remaining food is vegetable fibre (from rice or wheat husks for example). We now know that it is very important to have this fibre in our diet to keep the digestive system working well. Unfortunately it is fashionable in many places to eat highly polished or 'white' rice. Many people also eat flour and grains which have been milled in a factory. They even sell their whole grain crops which they have grown themselves, to buy these refined foods. This can lead to poor health. Our bodies need the whole grain to keep them working properly.

In the **mouth**, teeth cut up the food. Saliva is added from the salivary glands. The saliva makes the food slippery and begins to act on it chemically. The food is then swallowed and goes down the **oesophagus** or gullet (see diagram) into the **stomach**. The stomach is like a bag which can stretch. It can hold all the food which has been eaten during a meal. The stomach is muscular.

Some Teaching Suggestions

When reading this part of the chapter, refer also to chapter 8. You will find in chapter 8 ideas about how to tell stories, and how to use songs and drama in teaching. The following are some activities which you could do with the children:

Food around

Children could make a list of:
- foods which can be found in the market
- foods which can be seen in the garden
- foods which can be seen in the shop
- foods which can be seen on bushes and trees

Can they draw and label some of these foods? Or say whether they are GO, GROW, GLOW or STAPLE foods? (See earlier in this chapter.)

Make a cook book with the children. Children could watch their mothers cooking meals at home. They could note down on a piece of paper what she does. They could make a drawing of what she does. Groups of children (or the whole class) could put these pieces of paper together with a string to make little books. You could use these books to talk with the children about the foods which they like, the value of the food which they eat, and so on.

Make food cards with the children. Write a list of the common foods in your area. Now cut out small pieces of card about 4 cm × 5 cm. Write one food from your list on each card. Draw a picture of the food too. Older children might be able to help with this. The cards might look like this:

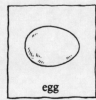 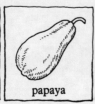

| egg | papaya | pineapple |

The children have to sort the cards into groups such as STAPLE, GO, GROW, GLOW foods. (You can use different names for the groups of foods if you wish such as **energy, growth, protection** foods.) A list might include some of the following:

Banana	GO
Beans (long)	GROW/GLOW
Beans (soya)	GROW
Bread	GO
Cabbage	GLOW
Carrot	GLOW
Cassava	STAPLE
Cheese	GROW
Chicken	GROW
Coconut	GO
Corn	GO
Egg	GROW
Fat	GO
Fish	GROW
Goat	GROW
Guava	GLOW
Green leaves	GLOW
Lemon	GLOW
Liver	GROW
Mango	GLOW
Meat	GROW
Milk	GO/GROW/GLOW
Orange	GLOW
Papaya	GLOW
Peanuts	GO/GROW
Peas	GROW
Pineapple	GLOW
Plain flour	GO
Potato	GO
Rice	STAPLE
Seaweed	GLOW
Shell fish	GROW
Sorghum	STAPLE
Sugar	GO
Spinach	GLOW
Tomato	GLOW
Yam	STAPLE

They could make their groups of cards on the floor or on a desk like this:

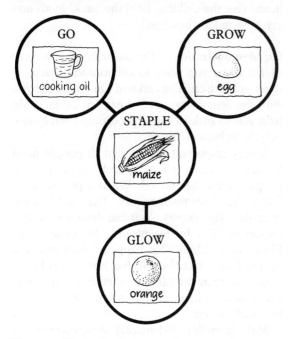

They could check their own groups against your list. Using the food cards, children can put foods together to make a balanced meal, and they can continue this for a whole day's meals. If there is school lunch, ask children if it is balanced (one food from each group). If not, can they suggest what would make it better? Children could then plan meals for a whole week.

The cost of food

Get the children to consider the cost of food. Often the cost of food is important. Get them to consider how cheaply they can make a balanced meal. Which food is the cheapest? Which food is the cheapest in each food group?

Take the children on a trip to the market and the local store. **In the market** get them to find out how much food in each of the food groups costs. You could divide the class into the food groups

and make each group responsible for finding out the cost of foods in that group only. On return to the classroom, children can learn from the other groups the cost of their foods.

In the store get the children to look for one item each. For example, they might look for margarine which they need for energy and vitamins. They might also look for 'junk foods' such as lolly water (fizzy drinks), and crisps which have little value for health. In the classroom, add the good food prices to the food groups. Take the junk foods and get children to work out how much good food they could have had for a bottle of fizzy drink or a bag of crisps etc.

1 bottle = 1 egg + pumpkin + 2 oranges + 1 slice
coke   leaves   bread

Teaching techniques

Tell stories to the children. Can you make up stories to emphasise some of the main ideas about food from this chapter? Here are some suggestions but perhaps you can develop them:
- 'A day in the life of my hands'. Make up a story about what hands touch during a typical day. The story could stress the point that hands should be clean if food is handled.
- 'Breast is best'. The story should emphasise that breast milk makes healthy babies.
- 'Good food'. Tell a story about two families. One family has plenty of good food, a mixed diet, and the mother feeds her babies breast milk. Another family has a poor diet and the babies are fed on bottles. The poorly fed family learns from the healthy family.

Act plays with the children. Children enjoy acting little plays. You could make up plays about:

- Food being digested in the body. (Perhaps the majority of the children in the class could be the food pipe. Others could be the food which is broken down into simpler substances and absorbed into the blood . . . .)
- A poor family where the mother has become blind in one eye. One of her children learns in school about the importance of vitamin A. She tells the family but they do not believe her. Eventually, she convinces them.

Check advertisements. In chapter 7, you will read how advertisements are used to influence us to buy things. They are often used to persuade us to buy certain foods and drinks.

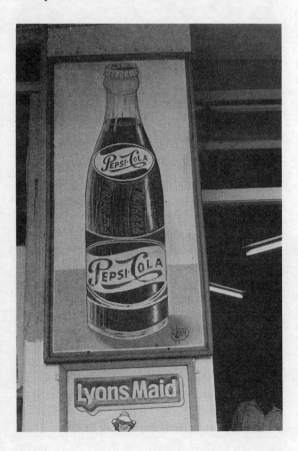

Can the children collect advertisements? Make a class display. Discuss the advertisements with them. Can the children label the 'junk' foods and say how much they cost?

Do demonstrations. Demonstrations are very useful when you want to communicate facts or ideas to children. The children can often help you with the demonstration. For example, they could help you to make a model food tube from boxes, polythene bags etc.

A very important idea is that **ill people need to eat**. In some places, people think that ill people should be starved. When a person has a fever, they use much energy. They need to eat to replace this energy. You can demonstrate this important idea by means of a kerosene lamp. Show the children what happens when you turn up the flame. Get them to feel how much hotter it is. Ask them to tell you whether it uses more fuel when the flame is high or low. Compare this to a sick person.

Make a model food market somewhere in the classroom. The children could make models of fruits and other foods, or bring the real food into the classroom. Use the market to discuss points about healthy eating.

When you talk about food groups, bring examples of the foods to school. Do demonstrations if possible. They will bring your teaching to life.

Discussions and talks can be useful. Use special incidents to discuss food with the children. Talk about the food eaten at religious festivals, for example. Discuss eating habits within the family. Are there any vegetarians in the class? Why are they vegetarian?

Can the health worker from the clinic talk to the children? She could explain how they weigh babies to check that they are growing properly. She can explain the importance of a good mixed diet.

Sing songs with the children.

Let's eat good food every day, every day, every
day,
Let's eat good food every day,
To keep our bodies healthy.

Let's eat three mixed meals a day, every day,
every day,
Let's eat three mixed meals a day,
To keep our bodies healthy.

This is just one possible song about food. Can
you make up any more based on the ideas about
food and eating in this chapter? Could you use
them in the plays suggested above?

Use CHILD-to-Child activities

Older children at school could help their mothers
by taking younger brothers and sisters (under
five) to the clinic. Young children should be
weighed regularly to check that they are growing
properly. Their weight should increase every
month.

Older children in the school could help to
weigh and measure the height of younger children in the school.

Do any children have younger brothers and
sisters who are ill? Explain to them that ill children must eat. They must eat often. When
illness is over, they should eat **more** than usual.
Encourage them to help their families in this
way.

Can older children at school plan meals for
their younger brothers and sisters? Show them
that, in addition to the STAPLE food, small
children need a concentrated GO food, a GROW
food (such as beans or peas or dahl), and a
GLOW food (such as leafy vegetables). Remember
that young children need to eat often. Their
stomachs are small.

Grow good food at school

Vegetables
The best vegetables to grow are those which have
dark green leaves. These give vitamin A and
some iron, and a small amount of protein. Leaves
which have good health value are pumpkin, sweet
potatoes, beans, peas and baobab leaves. They
can be eaten as a vegetable on their own or
dried, powdered, and mixed with baby gruel.
Cassava leaves are more nutritious than the root
and so provide a cheap, good food. Even if
children eat a lot of sweet potatoes and cassava,
remember that this alone will not provide a
healthy meal. Remember, also, that small
children cannot eat much of these as they are too
bulky.

Beans
Beans are vegetables which are a good source of
protein or body building foods. They are very
cheap. Soya beans are especially high in protein
but they are difficult to prepare except in a
community that is used to them. If they sprout
before cooking, they are higher in vitamins. Baby
food can be made from them by cooking them
well, peeling them and mashing them. It is a
good idea to soak beans in water for a few hours
before cooking them to soften them. This will
save cooking time and fuel. Throw away the
liquid in which you have soaked them before
adding more liquid for cooking.

Chickens
Many families keep chickens. They are a good
source of animal protein. The eggs are also a
good and cheap source of protein, which can be
mixed with other foods for children.

Fruit
Some people throw away fruit or feed it to
animals. This is a waste as fruit can give us
vitamins. Some people feed papaya to animals. If
you grow fruit make sure that your family eats
some of it too! Citrus fruits, like oranges, limes
and lemons are high in vitamin C. They can
make a good snack during the day, particularly if
you are thirsty!

Does your school have room for planting food crops? Does the school have a garden? If the school is in the town, see if you can obtain some big pots or use a part of the school compound. Of course, not all teachers will know about gardening. If you come from a rural area, you may know a lot. If you do not know very much, perhaps people who live near the school can help. Parents who have children in the school are particularly likely to help.

With food from the school garden or food which the children bring, can you plan a class or school feast occasionally? Are the parents willing to help? The children could help in the planning of the feast and in the preparation.

What do the children eat at break time? Do local traders sell snacks to the children? Is milk provided by the school? Can the children explain where these foods come from and how they get to the school?

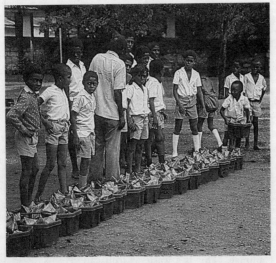

Children in a Kenyan school receive a daily milk packet

Recognising malnutrition

Look at these two children shown below. One eats good food. One is not well nourished. How can you tell?

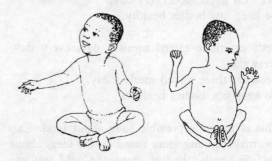

How can you recognise malnutrition? How can we help children to recognise malnutrition? One very useful way is to make the strip shown on page 73. Show the children how it works on one of their own arms (although they will be too old to give a true reading).

Peter is in the red
(his arm is too thin)

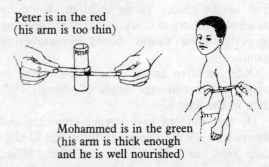

Mohammed is in the green
(his arm is thick enough
and he is well nourished)

Then get the children to practise on bamboos, bottles, or anything of the same shape. They could use the wrists of other children in the class. When they have learned how to do this, ask them to use the strip on their brothers and sisters below the age of five. Help them to keep proper records. In class, note down what children tell you. You could get them to draw a bar graph to show if there is a problem of malnutrition in the community.

too thin red area	healthy green area
///	//

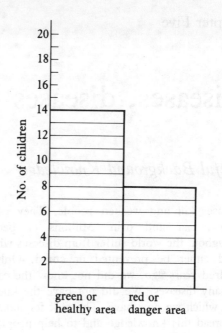

Chapter Five

Diseases, diseases

Useful Background Knowledge

Diseases kill and weaken people. They cause misery, fear and pain. Millions of people throughout the world suffer from diseases which could either be prevented or cured. Only a hundred years ago, we did not know the cause of many diseases. We did not have the knowledge which we now have. The task for today is to spread this knowledge and to help people to understand what can be done to prevent or cure disease.

In this chapter, the physical causes of disease will be explained. However, it is important to remember what we said in chapter 3 about the causes of disability (see page 50). There is often a chain of causes behind the physical cause. People often see this chain of causes from their own point of view. For instance:

- Perhaps as teachers, we consider that the main cause of disease is **ignorance**. We believe that people should be educated so that they understand good health practices.
- A health worker may consider that the main problem is **lack of a good water supply**. Without clean water, it is difficult for people to avoid disease.
- A person in a small village may believe that his sickness is due to **witchcraft** or because he has made a god angry.

When people are poor, there is often a cycle of poverty and disease. Poverty creates the conditions in which disease can flourish. Disease weakens people so that it is difficult for them to tackle the poor conditions in which they live.

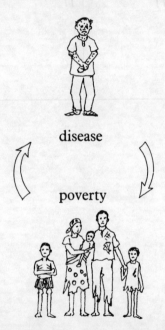

disease

poverty

Thus there is a cycle of poverty and disease. People often find it hard to escape from this cycle. Help children to understand that there is a combination of causes behind disease. Try to find out the main diseases in your area. Several important diseases are described in this chapter. Not all of them will be important where you live and teach. Concentrate on the most common ones and try to understand the chain of causes. It may be more effective to tackle some underlying causes rather than the direct cause.

Types of disease and their causes

There are two main types of disease. **Non-infectious** diseases do not spread from a sick person to a healthy person. They are not caught. **Infectious** diseases are spread from person to person. A healthy person can catch the disease from the infected person.

Non-infectious diseases

The table gives some examples of non-infectious diseases and their causes.

Immediate cause	Example
something wears out or goes wrong in the body	rheumatism, heart disease, arthritis, cancer, stroke, cataract of eye
something from outside harms or troubles the body	accident, snake bite, cough from smoking, allergy, asthma
lack of right kind or amount of food	malnutrition, goitre, anaemia, pellagra
something goes wrong with the mind	mental illness
people are born with a particular problem	harelip, epilepsy, mental handicap

It is difficult to prevent some of these diseases. However, diseases caused by accidents, smoking, and malnutrition can be prevented. These problems are discussed elsewhere in this book.

Infectious diseases

In the rest of this chapter, we will discuss infectious diseases. These diseases are mainly caused by tiny organisms called **bacteria**, **viruses**, and **fungi**. These are called germs. Some diseases are also caused by **parasites** which live either in or on the body.

Bacteria (singular-bacterium)

Although certain bacteria cause important diseases in man, many are harmless or beneficial. For example, bacteria play an important part in the carbon and nitrogen cycles of nature and in the recycling of nutrients. We also use bacteria to make certain foods such as cheese and yoghurt. Some bacteria live in the large intestine and are important for the digestion of food in the gut.

Bacteria are very small living organisms. One million would fit on the head of a pin. Under a high-powered microscope, it is possible to see their structure. There are several different kinds which are illustrated here. The diagrams show the bacteria enormously magnified. This is how they would appear under a high power microscope.

Spherical bacteria (*cocci*)

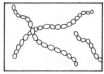
Streptococcus (some throat infections)

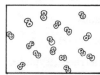
Diplococcus (pneumonia)

Rod shaped bacteria (*bacilli*)

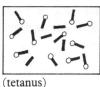
(tetanus)

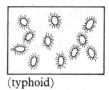
(typhoid)

Spiral shaped bacteria (*spirochaete*)

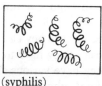
(syphilis)

Bacteria can reproduce very quickly, especially in the warm, moist, nourishing situation found between the cells of the human body. A single bacterium can divide every twenty minutes into two new bacteria. This is a very fast reproductive rate. We can grow many bacteria on food substances.

They produce toxins (poisons) as a result of their living processes. The toxins can cause disease in the person.

The table below shows some important bacterial diseases and how they are spread:

Disease	How it is spread
tuberculosis	through the air (coughing)
pneumonia	through the air (coughing)
some kinds of diarrhoea	dirty hands, water, flies
tetanus	dirty wounds
boils, sores	direct contact (touch)
gonorrhoea, syphilis	sexual contact

Antibiotics are the main kind of medicine which can be used to cure bacterial diseases. However, some diseases have become resistant to antibiotics so that new ones constantly have to be developed.

Viruses
Viruses are much smaller than bacteria. Very approximately, one million viruses could fit inside one bacterium! They are so small that they cannot be seen through a normal microscope. A special microscope, called an electron microscope, has to be used. They cannot be grown on food like bacteria. They have to be grown inside living cells. They have various shapes. Some are rod-shaped while others have more complex shapes.

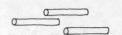
rod shaped virus

a virus with a more complex shape

Remember that these diagrams show viruses magnified enormously. A typical virus is only one ten-thousandth of a millimetre in diameter.

Like bacteria, they can reproduce very quickly. They attach themselves to a living cell. Part of the virus passes into the cell. New viruses are then formed inside the cell which eventually bursts releasing the new viruses. These, in turn, can infect other cells. The table below shows some important viral diseases and how they are spread:

Disease	How it is spread
measles, chickenpox, mumps, polio, colds, influenza ('flu), viral diarrhoea	through the air (by coughing, flies etc.)
rabies	animal bites
warts	touch

Antibiotics do not cure diseases caused by viruses. Although there are no medicines which can cure viral diseases, vaccinations are effective against some (such as polio and measles).

Other causes of disease
Bacteria and viruses are the main organisms which cause disease. However, some other diseases are caused by parasites and fungi. Fungi cause 'athlete's foot' and ringworm both of which are itchy irritations of the skin. Some internal parasites cause important diseases (see table on page 85):

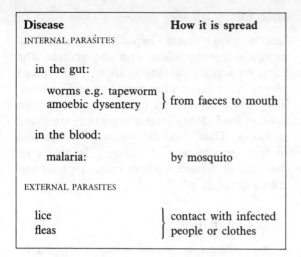

Disease	How it is spread
INTERNAL PARASITES	
in the gut:	
worms e.g. tapeworm amoebic dysentery }	from faeces to mouth
in the blood:	
malaria:	by mosquito
EXTERNAL PARASITES	
lice fleas }	contact with infected people or clothes

The spread of disease

Diseases enter the body either through the skin or through body openings.

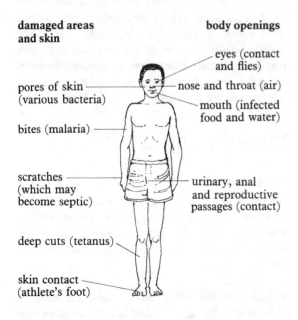

damaged areas and skin

- pores of skin (various bacteria)
- bites (malaria)
- scratches (which may become septic)
- deep cuts (tetanus)
- skin contact (athlete's foot)

body openings

- eyes (contact and flies)
- nose and throat (air)
- mouth (infected food and water)
- urinary, anal and reproductive passages (contact)

Hookworm, bilharzia, malaria, rabies, tetanus, and boils are examples of diseases where the disease-causing organisms enter through the skin. Sometimes, as in malaria and rabies, the disease enters due to the bite of an animal. Many diseases enter through body openings; namely the nose, mouth, eyes, anus and reproductive organs (penis or vagina). Eye diseases, colds, diseases which are spread through food and water, and venereal diseases are typical examples.

As indicated in the tables above, infectious diseases spread from one person to another through the following ways:

- air
- water
- food
- bodily contact
- insects
- animals
- faeces

Air

Colds, coughs, influenza, and tuberculosis are typical diseases which are spread through the air. The viruses or bacteria are spread when the person coughs or sneezes. In crowded places, the organisms can easily pass from one person to another so that the disease spreads rapidly. Remember not to cough or sneeze without covering your mouth and nose. People with tuberculosis should **never** spit on the floor.

Water

Some very important diseases are spread through water. They are often diseases which affect the intestine such as cholera, dysentry, and typhoid. Certain other diseases such as bilharzia are also spread by water. The disease organisms may pass out with the urine and faeces into water. If the

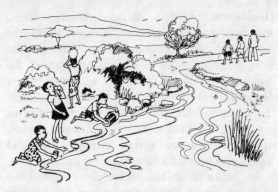

water is not treated and if people drink it, then the disease will enter their bodies. In this way, the disease is passed on.

Food

Disease may also be spread through food. Disease organisms may reach food through flies or on dirty hands. They can reproduce quickly using the food itself as a rich source of nutrient. When people eat the food, they are infected. Food is likely to become infected if:

- it is washed in water containing the disease organism
- it is touched by hands infected with germs from faeces
- flies land on the food
- it is touched by hands which have septic wounds on them

This is why food, especially meat, should be thoroughly cooked to kill germs. Hands should always be clean when food is prepared.

Bodily contact

Venereal diseases (mainly gonorrhoea and syphilis) are spread through sexual contact. They pass very easily from one person to another. In some countries, they are a most serious problem. Ringworm and athelete's foot are spread through contact (often via clothes, or via the floor).

Insects

Insects spread several important diseases. The mosquito spreads yellow fever and malaria. The tsetse fly spreads sleeping sickness. Fleas spread plague and typhus. Flies spread several diseases. They may carry faeces on their feet and then land on food. Many disease organisms are found in faeces. Thus, food can become infected and in turn, people become infected. In this way, flies spread diseases such as polio, typhoid and food poisoning.

Other animals

A most dangerous disease which is spread by dogs (and other animals such as foxes, wolves, jackals and cats) is rabies. An animal which is infected may act strangely, foams at the mouth, and may go mad, biting anything or anyone. A person who is bitten may become infected. The person becomes unable to swallow, especially to drink water, and becomes mentally ill. If a person is bitten by a rabid animal he must get medical help immediately. This consists of a series of anti-rabies injections. Once the disease begins in a person, it is impossible to save his life. Certain other less important diseases (such as viral throat infections from dogs) are also spread by animals.

Preventing disease

The body has its own natural system of defences against disease. The skin, for example, acts as a barrier to germs, preventing them from getting inside the body. However, if germs do enter the body, they meet another defence system and the following happens:

- Some of the white blood cells can actually 'swallow' bacteria (rather like an amoeba eats its food).

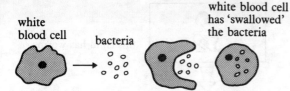

white blood cell   bacteria   white blood cell has 'swallowed' the bacteria

- The body immediately recognises when something 'foreign' has entered it. Foreign substances are called antigens. They stimulate the body to make substances called antibodies which fight the antigen. Antibodies are quite specific to a particular antigen. For example, the antibodies against measles have no effect on the polio virus.

- The antibodies remain even after the person has recovered from the disease. Thus, for many diseases, a person will not suffer from the disease again if he has already had it once. The antibodies provide protection. However, for some diseases, such as the common cold, there are so many different viruses that it is impossible to have resistance to them all. This is why colds are such a common form of illness.

Vaccination

Vaccination helps the body's natural defences against disease, and prevents people from catching certain diseases. Different vaccines work in different ways. These are listed below:

- Toxins (poisons) produced by the bacteria of a certain disease are made harmless. When they are injected into a person, they stimulate the production of antibodies. The diphtheria vaccine works in this way.

- Sometimes the bacteria may be killed and then injected. Again, this stimulates the production of antibodies but does not harm the person. The whooping cough vaccine works in this way.

- A weak and therefore harmless strain of a virus or bacteria may be used as a vaccine. It stimulates the body to produce antibodies which are also effective against the harmful strain of the virus or bacteria. The BCG vaccine against tuberculosis (TB) works like this.

Vaccination of children is particularly important. It can prevent them from catching serious diseases. Parents and health centres need to keep careful records of the vaccinations which children have had. Below is a typical vaccination schedule. There may be variations on this in some countries.

It is important that children receive the full course of vaccinations. Children and adults can also be given these vaccinations at other times but it is important to check details with qualified health workers. All adults, for example, should be protected against tetanus (lockjaw) which is provided by a course of three injections, injection number two following six weeks after the first and the third injection being given three years later.

Disease/vaccine	Schedule	How vaccine given
polio	at 3 months, 4 months, 5 months	by drops in a sugar lump or drops in mouth
'Triple vaccine' against diphtheria, whooping cough, tetanus	at 3 months, 4 months, 5 years	injections
'BCG' against tuberculosis	single injection at birth or any time after	injection – normally to skin of right shoulder
measles	at nine months	single injection

Vaccinations may also be given in certain countries against yellow fever, cholera, typhus and German measles.

Other ways of preventing disease

Vaccinations are an important method for preventing people from catching diseases. However, they are not the only method. Disease can be prevented by **personal and public hygiene**.

In chapter 2, the importance of personal hygiene was stressed. In this chapter, the spread of diseases has been explained. It follows that if we can stop diseases from spreading, people are less likely to catch them.

Diseases of the gut are often spread through people's stools (or faeces) and improved hygiene can reduce spread of these diseases. Diarrhoea, worms, cholera, typhoid and polio are spread in this way. The pictures here show how diarrhoea and worms are spread.

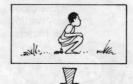

this child has worms

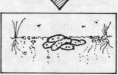

the faeces with the worm eggs go into the soil

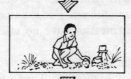

another child plays in the soil

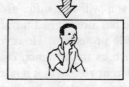

the child sucks his fingers and becomes infected

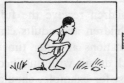

Ali has diarrhoea

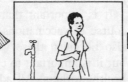

he forgets to wash his hands

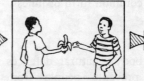

he gives Yakuba some food

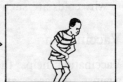

Yakuba now has diarrhoea

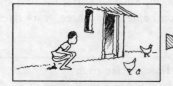

Mary has diarrhoea

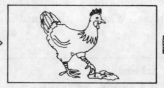

the chicken walks in the dirt

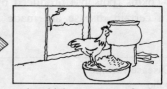

the chicken steps on food

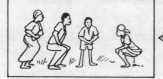

the family gets diarrhoea

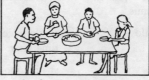

the family eat the food

Here are some important points to remember about preventing disease through personal and public hygiene. Many are discussed in more detail elsewhere in this book but they are summarised here. It is important to teach these ideas to children.

REMEMBER

- Wash hands with soap: in the morning, after using toilet and before eating food.

- Wash hands after handling soil.

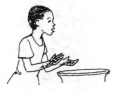

- Wash body often and look after teeth.

- Wear shoes outside if hookworm is common. (Hookworms enter through the soles of the feet.)

- Don't let children and babies eat soil or faeces.

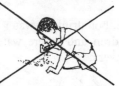

- Keep animals out of the house as far as possible. Don't let dogs lick children.

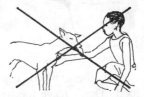

- Delouse the family often. Lice and fleas spread disease.

- Keep the area around the house and school clean. Clear up the faeces of dogs and animals.

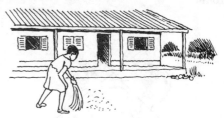

- Don't spit on the floor. Cover your nose and mouth with a handkerchief or cloth when you cough or sneeze.

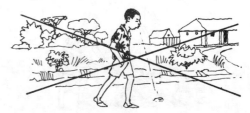

- People with tuberculosis, coughs and colds should, so far as possible, eat separately from others.
- If possible, boil drinking water – especially for small children and where water comes from holes or rivers.

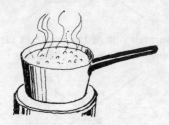

- Remember that flies spread disease. Keep them off food. Don't leave food scraps lying around. Keep food covered.

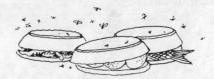

- Don't eat food which has gone bad. Throw it away. Wash fruit which has fallen to the ground.

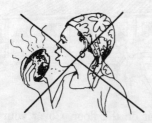

- Bury or burn rubbish.

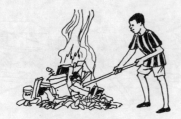

- Make a pit latrine (see page 185) and ensure that people use it. Don't urinate or defaecate in streams or rivers.

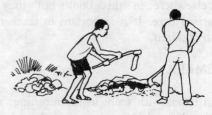

- Protect children from disease. Make sure that they get enough food. Well-nourished children can resist disease more easily than those who have been poorly-fed.
- Sick children should, if possible, sleep away from those who are well.
- Keep children clean. Cut fingernails short.

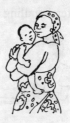

- Take particular care with babies. Remember . . . 'breast is best'.

(See also chapter 11 for ideas about encouraging public hygiene in the community.)

Some important diseases

Diarrhoea

Diarrhoea is the name given to the condition where a person produces frequent, watery stools (faeces). The person may also vomit and have cramps in the stomach. The stools smell different from normal stools. Diarrhoea is caused by germs which enter a person's mouth (from dirty water, for example). There are many different causes of diarrhoea: bacteria, viruses, malaria, food poisoning, eating unripe fruit etc. However, most diarrhoea is caused by infection and poor nutrition.

In many places, diarrhoea kills large numbers of babies and young children. It is often the most common cause of death in children between the ages of six months and two years. It is more likely to kill a baby who is malnourished.

The main reason why children die of diarrhoea is that they lose water from their bodies. They become dehydrated. When a baby becomes dehydrated, the soft spot (fontanelle) on the top of the head sags. On page 100, there is an idea for a demonstration to show why this happens. The following are also signs of dehydration:

- the child produces little or no urine (the urine is dark yellow)
- dry mouth
- sunken tearless eyes
- the skin loses its stretchiness (if you lift up the skin and can still see the fold after you have let go, then the child is dehydrated)

Making a special drink

The most important treatment for diarrhoea is to put water back into the body. The best way of doing this is to make up a special drink containing water, sugar, and salt. The water replaces the lost liquid. The sugar helps the salt and water to be absorbed by the intestine and provides energy for the body. The salt replaces that which is being lost from the body. The diagram illustrates how to make the drink.

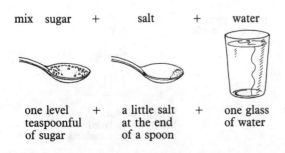

mix sugar + salt + water

one level + a little salt + one glass
teaspoonful at the end of water
of sugar of a spoon

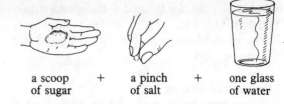

a scoop + a pinch + one glass
of sugar of salt of water

DON'T USE TOO MUCH SALT

In many countries of the world, a special plastic spoon is available. It looks like this:

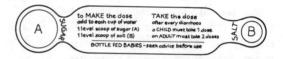

A SUGAR
to MAKE the dose
add to each cup of water
1 level scoop of sugar (A)
1 level scoop of salt (B)
BOTTLE FED BABIES - seek advice before use
TAKE the dose
after every diarrhoea
a CHILD must take 1 dose
an ADULT must take 2 doses
SALT B

It shows the correct amount of sugar and salt for each glass or cup. The drink should be no more salty than tears.

You should give the drink as soon as dehydration begins. A child should drink one glass for each stool passed. An adult should drink two.

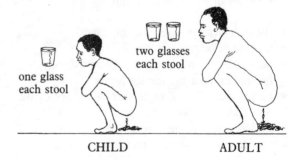

one glass each stool

two glasses each stool

CHILD   ADULT

Give the drink every two or three minutes if necessary, day and night, until the child urinates every two or three hours. Give the drink slowly, one teaspoon every five minutes. After drinking, the diarrhoea may increase. Don't worry. The child must drink as much liquid as he loses.

Use water which has been boiled and cooled to make the drink. In many places this can be difficult. Water which has been used to cook rice or vegetables can also be used as the special drink. You do not need to add sugar and salt in this case. Dilute tea (without milk) but with the sugar and salt can be used.

Other action to take

Children with diarrhoea should be given food if they can eat it without vomiting. The food will help them to fight the sickness. Don't give fatty or greasy foods, nor most raw fruit, nor highly seasoned foods.

Mothers should continue to breast feed babies who have diarrhoea. The milk replaces the liquid which they are losing and provides food.

Follow the suggestions made earlier in this chapter about preventing the spread of diarrhoea. Prevention is better than cure!

Warning signs

Often a child will recover from diarrhoea provided that he does not become dehydrated. Some diarrhoea is serious and it may not be possible for the child to recover without medical assistance. Take the child to the health clinic if he shows any of the following signs:

- the dehydration does not improve
- he cannot or will not drink
- he vomits so much that he cannot drink
- he makes no urine for six hours
- he has diarrhoea so often that he cannot drink one glass per stool
- he has blood in his stool
- the diarrhoea lasts for more than two days

Malaria

Malaria is an infection of the blood. The person has chills and a high fever. It is spread by mosquitos.

The parasites are passed from one person to another only by mosquitoes. An attack of malaria usually begins with a chill. The person shivers and shakes. Later, his temperature rises very high (often more than 40°C) for several hours. Finally the person begins to sweat and his temperature comes down. These attacks may occur every two or three days. However, in children, the pattern may not be like this. The disease is particularly dangerous in small children under the age of five. The child may become weakened by the repeated fevers. It may affect his brain, causing fever, fits, and death.

A medicine called **chloroquine** (it often has special brands names such as **nivaquine**) should be taken by a person with malaria. In can be taken in tablet form. If possible, seek advice from the health clinic.

Aspirin is not the medicine to treat malaria.
Aspirin may, however, reduce a person's fever.

Prevention

The most obvious method of preventing the disease is to prevent people from being bitten by mosquitos. Babies should sleep under a net if possible. Spraying by the public health authorities will help to reduce the number of mosquitoes. Mosquitoes breed in standing water. Get

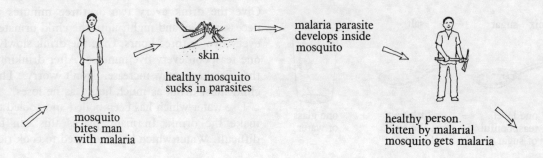

mosquito bites man with malaria

skin

healthy mosquito sucks in parasites

malaria parasite develops inside mosquito

healthy person bitten by malarial mosquito gets malaria

rid of places such as old pots, tins or ponds where water can lie, and in which mosquitoes can lay their eggs.

In the past, health education has often concentrated on killing mosquitos. However, there are other ways of controlling the disease. In places where malaria is common, people can take anti-malarial medicine. Many adults in areas where malaria exists have immunity or partial immunity to the disease. They do not need to take the drug. But children are not immune. The disease can be very dangerous for them. Thus children between three months and five years (and also pregnant women) who live in malarial areas should take the anti-malarial drug. Great care is necessary to ensure that the right dose is given. At the age of five, the medicine should not be stopped suddenly. The dose should be reduced gradually.

Tuberculosis (TB)

Tuberculosis is a serious disease. It affects many adults in developing countries, particularly those between fifteen and twenty-five. It affects people who are weak, poorly nourished, or those who live with people who have the disease. It can be dangerous for young children. **Thousands of people die from TB every year. Yet it can be cured. It is important to know the signs of TB and to treat it early.**

TB is caused by bacteria which attack the lungs and other parts of the body. The disease develops slowly. It makes people worse over a period of months or even years. The signs of TB are:

- a chronic cough, especially after waking up (chronic means that it has lasted for a long time)
- increasing weakness and getting thinner
- mild fever in the afternoon and sweating at night
- in the later stages, coughing blood (however, this stage may not be reached for 6–12 months; meanwhile, the person has got worse and infected others)

TB can pass very easily from one person to another.

Treatment

People who think that they have TB should go to the health clinic. Sputum (spit) can be examined under the microscope to check whether it contains the TB bacterium.

Often both injections and tablets are necessary. The injections may have to be given two or three times a week for two months. The tablets have to be taken for a long time, often for up to two years. Sometimes people stop taking the tablets because they feel better. This is very dangerous as the bacteria can become resistant to the medicine. They are no longer easy to kill with the medicine. Thus, it is most important that the full course of tablets is taken.

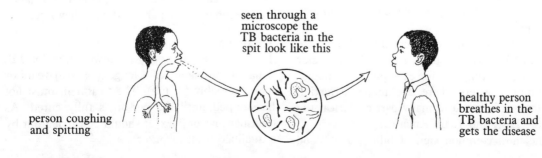

seen through a microscope the TB bacteria in the spit look like this

person coughing and spitting

healthy person breathes in the TB bacteria and gets the disease

Prevention

TB can be prevented if people are vaccinated. If one person in a house has TB, everyone else should be tested for the disease. Children should be vaccinated. If possible, the person should sleep separately from the others – especially children. An infected person should never spit on the floor and should cover his mouth when coughing. Treat TB early. If a child has had a cough for more than two weeks, take him to be tested at the nearest health clinic. The signs of the disease in children are different from those in the adult. The main signs in children are fever and getting thinner.

Remember

TB can be treated

treatment takes a long time

early treatment is important

relatives should be checked

BCG vaccinations prevent the disease

Bilharzia

Bilharzia is a worm which gets into the blood-stream through the skin. The worms settle in the blood vessels lining the bladder. They lay small eggs into the bladder. This causes blood to appear in the urine and this is often a sign of bilharzia. The eggs are passed out of the body in the urine. If the urine is passed into water, the eggs hatch and enter a certain kind of snail which lives in water. The worms develop further in the snail and when they come out they infect people by boring through the skin when people bathe in infected water. Thus the cycle continues (see page 95).

The people who most often catch the disease are farmers who have to spend much time in water channels, planting rice for example. The disease is common where there are major irrigation schemes. It is found in many part of Africa, the Middle East, and Latin America.

The most common **sign** of bilharzia is blood in the urine. An infected person may have pain low down in the abdomen. Sometimes the kidneys are damaged. In severe cases, people may die of the disease.

Treatment

Bilharzia can be treated by giving certain tablets. The tablets often have unpleasant side effects. They should only be given by experienced health workers or doctors.

Prevention

The best method of prevention is to stop the spread of the disease. **People should never urinate in or near water.** They should urinate in latrines. In some places, there are major programmes to kill snails. (Copper sulphate or lime is added to the water to kill the snails.)

Leprosy

Leprosy is not one of the killer diseases. However, it does cause much fear and super-stition (false beliefs). It develops very slowly – even more slowly than TB. It damages the nerves in the arms and legs. It is not as infectious as TB, and is very difficult to catch. It can be cured. People who are taking the correct treatment are not infectious. They do not have to go away from their own homes to take the treatment.

The **signs** of leprosy vary. Often the first main sign is a patch of pale or thickened skin. There may be a loss of feeling (numbness) in the skin patch, or in the hands or feet. People may burn themselves while cooking because they cannot feel pain. In advanced cases, the feet and hands may become partly paralysed and claw-like.

Treatment

This does exist for leprosy. However, as for TB, it has to be taken for a long time (two years or more; possibly for life). The treatment must not be stopped until the person is fully cured. As treatment is complex, it should be carried out by a qualified health worker.

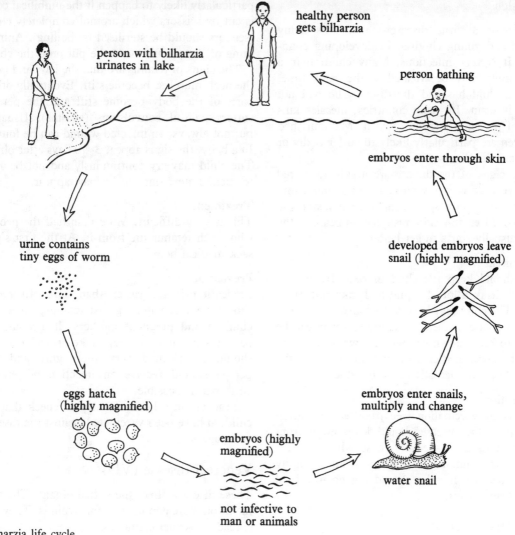

person with bilharzia
urinates in lake

healthy person
gets bilharzia

person bathing

embryos enter through skin

urine contains
tiny eggs of worm

developed embryos leave
snail (highly magnified)

eggs hatch
(highly magnified)

embryos (highly
magnified)

embryos enter snails,
multiply and change

not infective to
man or animals

water snail

Bilharzia life cycle

People who have the disease must be very careful to protect their hands and feet against damage (by cutting, bruising or burning). Damage is likely because they may not be able to feel pain. They should wear shoes. They should check their hands and feet carefully every day. If there is an open sore on them, they should be particularly careful to keep it clean and at rest until it is healed. They should not smoke.

> **Remember**
> With early treatment and care of limbs, the deformities of leprosy need not happen.
> Leprosy is a disease which can be cured.
> It is caused by a germ, like other diseases.
> People have not done anything wrong to catch it.
> They do not have to be sent away and isolated from other people.

Measles

Measles is a virus disease which kills many babies and young children in developing countries. It is very infectious. Many children in a community may be affected at the same time. Once a child has had the disease, he will not catch it again. In many countries, measles kills 10% of the children who catch it. Malnourished children are particularly likely to suffer badly or die from the disease.

The **signs** of the disease are a skin rash, red sore eyes, fever, runny nose, a cough, and a sore throat (tiny white spots can be seen inside the throat). After the skin rash has appeared, the child usually starts to get better.

Treatment

You should keep the child in bed. He or she should drink a lot of liquid and take nutritious food. The child may have to be coaxed to eat and drink because of the sore mouth. Aspirin can be given to bring down temperature when the fever is high. Local medicines should not be put in the eyes. They can actually cause blindness.

Prevention

This is by vaccination (see page 87). Children who have the disease should keep away from other children – especially those who have TB or are malnourished. Children from a family which has had measles should not go to school for fourteen days.

Tetanus (Lockjaw)

Tetanus is a deadly disease. It is caused by bacteria which live in the soil, especially soil which contains the faeces of animals. If the tetanus germs enter a cut or wound, the person may catch the disease. Deep or dirty wounds are particularly dangerous (for example wounds from animal bites, dirty needles, barbed wire or cuts from thorns).

New-born babies may also catch the disease through the umbilical cord stump. This is particularly likely to happen if the umbilical cord is cut by scissors which are not completely clean (scissors should be sterilised by boiling). Animal dung or dirt should never be put onto the cord.

The **signs** of tetanus are that the jaw, and later the neck muscles, become stiff. Eventually other parts of the body become stiff and the person suffers painful convulsions (spasms). Usually, but not always, an infected wound can be found. In a baby, the signs appear 3–10 days after birth. The child may cry continuously and not be able to suck. Later, signs of lockjaw appear.

Treatment

This is very difficult. More than half the people who catch tetanus die from it. At the first sign, seek medical help.

Prevention

Prevention is far easier than cure. Everyone should be vaccinated against tetanus, especially children and pregnant mothers. If a wound is particularly dirty or deep, take special care. It should be cleaned very thoroughly and the person should receive an injection of tetanus anti-toxin if possible.

Teachers in school can help to check that all children have been vaccinated against the disease (see page 87).

Venereal disease (VD)

These diseases affect the sexual organs. The two mains ones are gonorrhoea and syphilis. They are spread by sexual contact.

Gonorrhoea

This does not kill people but it can cause much suffering and unhappiness.

The **signs** of the disease are vary according to sex. In men, there is often pain during urination. Pus may come from the penis. Sometimes, the man has a slight fever. In women, the signs are not so clear. A woman may have some lower abdominal pain during urination and a little pus may be produced from the vagina. (A pregnant woman with gonorrhoea may pass the infection on to the baby who gets a severe conjunctivitis which may cause blindness.) Later the woman may become sterile. Even though a woman may not appear to have the disease, she can still pass it on to her child or a sexual partner.

The **signs** of gonorrhoea in a man may show in two to five days (or up to three weeks) after sexual contact. In a woman, years may pass before she shows any signs. However, she may still be able to pass on the disease even if she shows no signs.

Treatment

This is by injection of penicillin or other antibiotics.

Syphilis

This, like gonorrhoea, is spread through sexual contact. The first **sign** of it is a sore like a pimple or blister which appears on the genital areas of men and women. In women, it may be on the inside of the vagina so that she does not know it is there. The sore is usually painless. It may appear 2–5 weeks after sexual contact with an infected person. It often goes away without treatment.

Treatment

Syphilis is an extremely serious disease. If it is not treated it can eventually cause damage to most organs of the body. It is treated by a course of penicillin injections.

AIDS

AIDS stands for **A**cquired **I**mmune **D**eficiency **S**yndrome. It is a most serious disease which has appeared only during the last few years. Its origin is not certain. In some countries, it is now a major cause of death among some groups of people.

It is caused by a virus which attacks the body's natural defence system. Some people who have the virus therefore get infections and illnesses which do not trouble healthy people.

People who carry the virus do not necessarily develop AIDS. But anyone who has the virus can pass it on to another person. Homosexuals (people who prefer sexual relationships with others of their own sex) are not the only ones who get AIDS although they are particularly at risk.

The AIDS virus is spread by:
- sexual intercourse with an infected person
- injection of infected blood

It is not spread by normal social contact such as shaking hands, social kissing or being physically close to other people.

At present there is no vaccine to protect people against AIDS. Nor is there any cure. However, there are ways to reduce its spread:
- the more sexual partners a person has, the more likely they are to have sex with an infected person
- using a condom (sheath) (see page 64) reduces the risk of AIDS and other venereal diseases
- any act which damages the penis, vagina, anus or mouth is dangerous, particularly if it causes bleeding
- drug users should not share needles or other equipment

Prevention of venereal disease

While this knowledge about VD may not be directly necessary for teaching primary school children, it is important that you, as a teacher, know how to prevent it:

- if you think you have any form of VD, get treatment immediately – do not have sex with anyone until at least three days after treatment is complete
- tell anyone else with whom you have had sexual contact to get treatment
- avoid brothels – prostitutes often have VD
- encourage people who have VD to get treatment

Some Teaching Suggestions

Essential knowledge and useful knowledge

It is not easy to learn and teach about diseases. There are many facts. The subject can easily become boring. How can we make it interesting to the children whom we teach? How can we help them to understand the ideas explained in the first part of this chapter? Perhaps we should begin by identifying for our own situation what is **essential knowledge** and what is **useful** knowledge.

Essential knowledge is the kind of knowledge which saves lives. It is knowledge about the main diseases which kill or maim people in your area. It is knowledge about how to prevent these diseases or to cure them. For example, it is essential knowledge to know how to treat diarrhoea in babies and young children.

Useful knowledge is the kind of knowledge which may not save lives directly, but which is relevant to the situation in which you live. For example, it is useful to know about the way in which diseases are spread and what causes them.

We must, of course, remember that the level of our teaching has to be adjusted to the age and ability of the children. 'Essential' knowledge for a teacher may not be 'essential' for a six-year-old child.

Question: Can you divide the knowledge in the Background Knowledge section of this chapter into essential and useful knowledge? Consider the situation of your own area, and the level of the children.

How we teach a subject is as important as **what** we teach. In teaching about diseases, we may feel

that the quickest way to teach these ideas is by traditional 'chalk and talk', thus:

- explain disease to the class
- write notes on the blackboard
- children copy notes in notebook
- children learn their notes
- test their knowledge about disease by a 'one-word-answer test out of ten'

There is a great temptation to teach in this way. We may consider that there are many facts to cover, the class is large and our responsibility great. However, it is not the only way to teach about disease. Chapter 8 explains in general the variety of methods which we can use in health education. Many of these methods you can use here.

Loosen up your approach!

Don't worry too much about covering all the facts about disease. It is unfortunate, but true, that we tend to forget facts easily. We are even more likely to forget those facts which we have learnt 'parrot-fashion' or which have little meaning for us. For much of the time spent in classrooms, teachers talk at children. It was probably the way that our teachers taught us. But it is not the only method of teaching. It is not necessarily the best method of teaching.

When you teach about disease, you are teaching about something which directly affects all the children in the class. Disease dramatically affects their lives. They know what it is like to be sick. They may also have experienced the death of people in their own family due to disease. Thus, this is a subject which will be interesting to children if you can relate your lessons to their lives. What does this mean in practice?

The following are some suggestions:

- Listen to the children. Let them tell you about the diseases which they have had or which have affected their families.
- Tell them that you don't know everything about disease. You will not lose their respect. Children will respect you more if they can see that you are honest and trying to help them.
- When you teach about disease, you will need to allow informal discussion. This does not mean that everyone talks at once. There has to be some discipline involved. Children have to learn to listen to what other children say. The teacher needs much skill to handle a discussion effectively. If children are to learn from it, it may be necessary to draw together what they have said at the end. You may need to summarise the key points on the board. Discussions often work better if the children can face each other. Take the children outside sometimes and let them sit in a U shape.

Teaching techniques

Stories can be used in different ways (see chapter 8). Can you make up some stories to help children understand about the causes of diseases and how we can prevent disease? Choose examples from your own area. Decide on the main message which you want the children to understand. Make sure that the message is emphasised in your story. You could make up stories about:

- A child whose baby sister has diarrhoea. He tells his mother about the special drink (see page 91) which he has learned about in school. His mother believes what he tells her (she lost another baby who had diarrhoea). She gives the drink and the baby recovers . . .
- A village where everyone gets bilharzia. A new teacher comes to the school. She explains both to the children and to the parents about the disease. The community make latrines and the children learn to use them. Gradually people get better . . .

- A girl's father who is coughing blood. She persuades him to go to the clinic. They give him some tablets to take. He begins to get better. He thinks he is cured, so stops taking the tablets. Then he begins to get worse again . . .
- A head-teacher who tries to organise a vaccination programme for a village. The head-man opposes the idea. However, the head-teacher wins support from other leading members of the community. The head-man is persuaded and eventually supports the idea enthusiastically . . .

Use everyday incidents. There will always be amongst the children, or their families, people who are suffering from disease. Use these incidents to make your teaching interesting and lively. For example:

- Have any of the children had an accident? What was the accident? What were the effects on that person? What help was given? Has the person recovered? (See chapter 6 for more ideas on this.)
- Have any of the children suffered from disease? What were the symptoms of the disease? How did the child feel? Did he take any medicine? Did he go to the health worker? What did the health worker say?
- Have any younger brothers or sisters suffered from disease? If so, what disease? Have the children in class used any of the ideas in chapter 9 about older children caring for younger children?

The children could carry out a survey of disease incidents in a younger class, over the period of a month. Each time a child is sick, a record is kept. Perhaps major illnesses might be:

- diarrhoea
- vomiting
- coughs
- colds

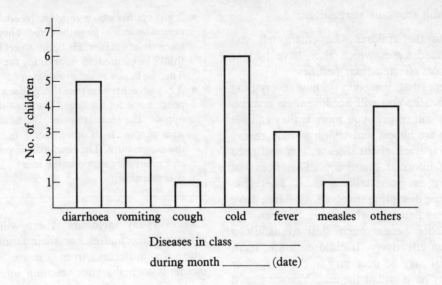

Diseases in class _____

during month _____ (date)

- fever
- measles
- other diseases (specify)

A bar chart could then be constructed, like the one shown above.

This activity could be related to the survey of diseases in the community by health scouts (see page 198).

Use dramatic demonstrations and examples. A dramatic demonstration or example can help children to understand about diseases and how they spread. Here are three ideas:

- **When you teach about the spread of disease through water** arrange the children in a circle. The first child washes his hands in a bowl of water. He then passes the bowl to the next who again washes his hands in the same water. The bowl is passed around the circle of children. When the bowl reaches the last child in the circle, ask him to drink the water! The children should realise that the water is now very dirty. (The water should not, of course, be drunk.) This demonstration can lead to a

good discussion about the need to keep drinking water clean. Water which is used for washing ourselves and our clothes should be kept separate from drinking water.

- **When you teach about dehydration of the body through diarrhoea** find a gourd or calabash (or even a tin can or plastic bottle). Make a hole at the base of the gourd and fit it with a plug of some kind (such as a cork or tightly folded piece of cloth). Make a hole at the top also. Fill up the gourd with water.

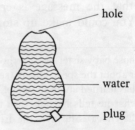

Explain that the water in the gourd represents the water in our bodies. Take out the cork. The water which drains out is like the liquid which is lost in diarrhoea. It must be replaced. More water must be added to the gourd – and to the person. You can make this model more realistic in several ways. Paint a face on the gourd. Make the hole at the top quite small, and cover it with a damp cloth. As the water drains out, the cloth sinks in. This is similar to the soft spot on a baby's head, the fontanelle, sinking in when the baby is dehydrated.

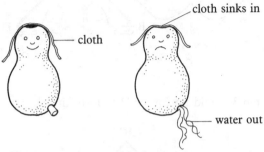

You can make small holes by the eyes so that the gourd baby who is dehydrated does not produce tears. You can make a hole in the front so that no urine is formed in a dehydrated gourd baby.

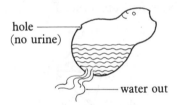

A hole could be made for the mouth. Fill up the gourd baby to the top. Now when the plugs are removed, the gourd baby both vomits and has diarrhoea. Water is lost even more quickly. Thus the children can learn that dehydration happens faster when vomiting occurs. Vomiting and diarrhoea together are therefore very dangerous.

- **Children can learn about the speed at which bacteria multiply** by using a chessboard and grains of rice. Put one grain on the first square, two on the second, four on the third, and so on. The number of grains will increase very rapidly. You could adjust this problem

to the level of the children. For example, you might ask older primary children to find out how many bacteria are produced in six hours assuming that bacteria divide every twenty minutes. (Thus, in six hours the bacteria will divide eighteen times. The number is therefore $2^{18} = 524\ 288$.)

The use of role-play in teaching about health to primary children is explained in more detail in chapter 8. Role-play can help children to understand and remember important ideas about diseases and their prevention. For example:

- They could act 'The Health Clinic'. Different children could pretend to have different diseases. Another child plays the health worker and tries to diagnose their symptoms. You can make the play more realistic by drawing marks on the children with a (washable) felt tip pen. Babies can be represented by dolls or cardboard cut-outs.
- They could act 'Preventing disease in our village'. The play could be based on a discussion at the village council or among family members at home.
- They could act 'Caring for younger brothers and sisters who are ill'. (Ideas for this are found in chapter 9.)

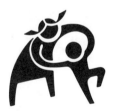

Remember that, in a role-play, there is no fixed script. The children behave and talk as they imagine real people would behave and talk in that situation. Children will need help, however, to give structure to the play and to get across the main ideas.

Making diarrhoea spoons

On page 91 is a plastic measuring spoon. This spoon measures the correct amount of sugar and salt for the 'special drink' for diarrhoea. However, it is made of plastic. It is not available everywhere. The spoon is useful as a **model**. It can be copied in many different ways. One way is to make paper cups of the correct size. This is something which children can do in class and which they will enjoy. You do not even need the plastic spoon as a model. If you use the dimensions shown below, the drink will be correct:

Step 1   Draw a square 6 cm × 6 cm on paper of a reasonably good quality. The square below is exactly the right size:

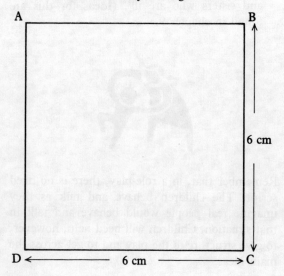

Step 2   Fold corner C across to corner A so that it now looks like this:

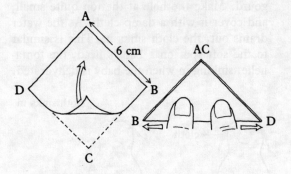

Step 3   Fold up corner D to form this shape:

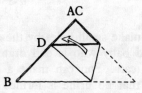

Step 4   Now fold up corner B:

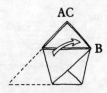

Step 5   This leaves two flaps at the top, A and C. Fold each flap back on itself:

Step 6 If you put your finger in the fold B–D, you have made a cup:

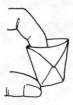

Step 7 This cup contains the correct amount of sugar for the special drink. Fill it level with the brim, thus:

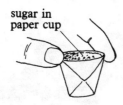

sugar in paper cup

You can also make a similar cup from a piece of paper 3 cm × 3 cm. The square below is exactly the right size.

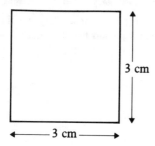

3 cm

← 3 cm →

Fill this cup with **salt**, level to the brim as for the **sugar**. Tip both the salt and the sugar into a medium-sized glass of water. Mix it well. If you want to know more exactly how much water to use, you can use the paper cup idea again to help you. Make a paper cup (dimensions 20 cm by 20 cm) using the same procedure as above. This will hold water for long enough to fill up a glass or container. Two paper cups of this size are the right amount. Make sure that the cups are filled to the brim. Use water which has previously been boiled and cooled.

A child should take one dose of this special drink after every attack of diarrhoea. An adult should take two doses after every diarrhoea. (See page 91.)

The photographs on the next page show children making and using these cups. This is an activity which they will enjoy. Get them to tell their parents about this idea.

There are many other ways by which you can calculate the correct amount of salt and sugar for the special drink. Holes can be drilled in wood. Tin cans and bottle tops, bamboos and teaspoons can all be used. Try out your own ideas.

DON'T USE TOO MUCH SALT

Invite the health worker to the school

The local health worker can tell your children about the common diseases in the area. Ask him to come to the school. Ask him to tell the children about the diseases which he treats. How can they be prevented? How can they be cured?

The health worker may know about diseases. He may not know very much about **how to teach children**. You may need to help him. Before the lesson, discuss with him what he will tell the children. You might suggest that he tells a story or does a demonstration. Make sure that his talk and visit fit in with your own teaching about disease. Remember that you may wish to invite him again to talk about other aspects of health. He may also wish to talk to other classes. Liaison with the head-teacher is therefore important.

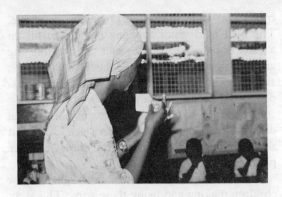
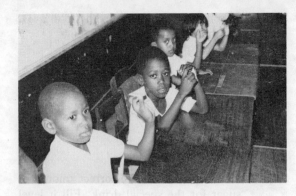
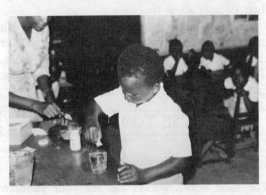
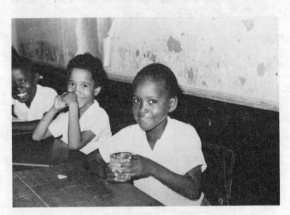

Children in a primary school in Mombasa, Kenya, learn how to make the paper cups. They use the cups to measure the right quantities of sugar and salt for the special drink when a person has diarrhoea.

Chapter Six

Safety first

Useful Background Knowledge

Accidents

In some schools, as many as two children will die each year because of accidents. For every child killed, about eighteen others will be seriously injured. MANY OF THESE ACCIDENTS NEED NOT HAPPEN.

Most accidents happen in these four places:

- at school
- in the home
- in the neighbourhood
- on the road

At school

Accidents at school often occur in the classroom. What dangers can you see in the classroom shown here?

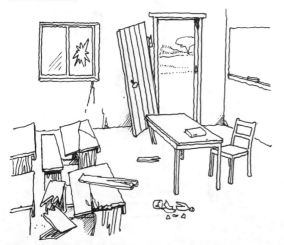

Sometimes accidents occur in the school grounds. You have probably seen places in school where accidents may occur. The picture illustrates some of the hazards occurring in school grounds.

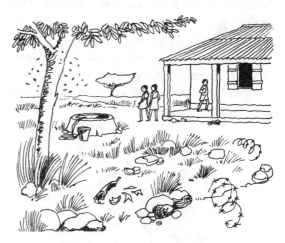

Children's behaviour sometimes causes accidents. What accidents can happen here?

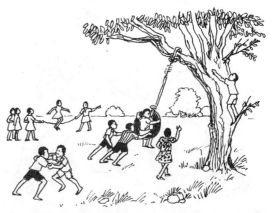

Prevention

You can prevent accidents at school by:

- mending broken chairs or desks
- getting rid of nails and splinters of wood which stick out
- making equipment safe
- clearing the ground of sharp objects
- cutting long grass
- helping children to understand what kind of behaviour will cause accidents

At home

Accidents in the home are very common. They include:

- Burns from cooking pots, open fires, cookers or lamps, electrical things, hot food, boiling water, steam, hot fat (scalds), strong acids or corrosives which damage the skin. (An example is the fluid from a car battery.)

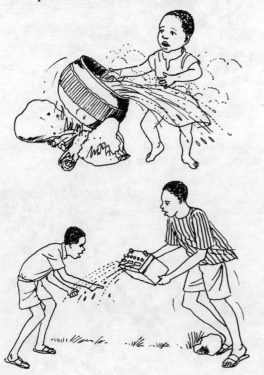

- Cuts from broken glass,
  rusty pins,
  rough wood,
  sharp knives

(Cuts can bleed a lot and become infected.)

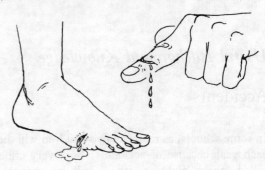

- Obstruction in breathing from swallowing small objects such as coins and buttons. (These objects block the passage of air to the lungs.)
- Poisoning. This is especially common in children who may eat or drink harmful substances. Children often eat tablets, such as aspirin or iron tablets, because they think that they are sweets. Sometimes harmful liquids such as methylated spirits or petrol are drunk.

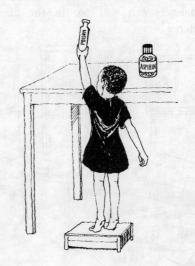

- Internal bleeding from swallowing sharp objects such as razor blades.
- Electric shock. This can occur if you touch a broken electrical appliance, a faulty plug or a switch. Your body comes into contact with the 'live' electric current. This causes the muscles of the body to contract. If the shock is severe, breathing stops, and the heart also stops. Death may result. Electric shock can occur if you repair electrical appliances when connected to the mains supply or if you touch electric wires outside the house. Electricity can be conducted through water. Never touch electric appliances, switches, or sockets, if you are wet. An electric shock when you are wet is even more dangerous.

Prevention

You can prevent accidents at home:

- put handles of cooking pots where children will not knock them over
- use a thick cloth when touching hot pots
- put fencing around fires and building them on clay piles
- clear the floor of broken glass and nails
- keep sharp knives and razors in a safe place, where children cannot reach them, such as in a drawer or cupboard or on a high shelf
- keep all medicine and poisons out of reach of children (lock them in a cupboard or trunk if you can, or put them on a high shelf)
- label all medicines and poisons clearly
- don't store kerosene or petrol in bottles

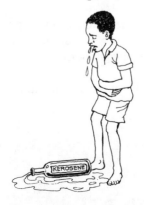

Preventing electric shocks

- Don't try to repair electrical appliances unless you know what you are doing. Never leave them plugged in when you are repairing them.

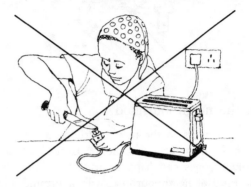

- Don't touch electrical wires outside the house.

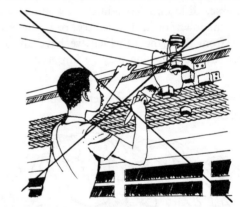

- Don't touch electrical appliances when your hands or feet are wet.

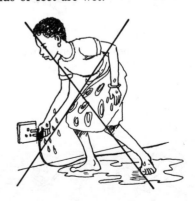

- Don't use plugs or wires which are damaged.

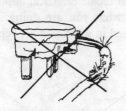

In the neighbourhood

Some dangers in the neighbourhood are similar to those in the school or home. Burns, cuts and broken bones can happen anywhere. However, the kind of neighbourhood will determine what are the most likely accidents. The dangers are, of course, different depending on whether you live in the town, or in the country, or by the sea. Apart from the dangers which we have already discussed, the following may be important:

- Poisoning from eating certain plants and berries.

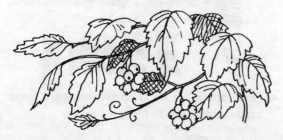

- Bites from animals. Dog bites may cause rabies. A bite from any animal may become infected. Snake bites can be a serious danger in some places.

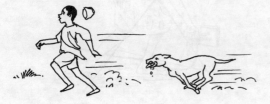

- Stings from bees and other insects. Jellyfish in the sea can also give nasty stings.

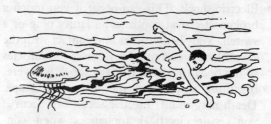

- Drowning. People can drown wherever there is open water (the sea, rivers, lakes, old quarries and even ponds).

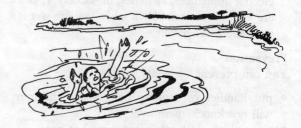

Prevention of neighbourhood accidents
- bury rubbish in pits
- always be very careful with fires
- cut long grass and clear areas where children often play
- do not eat fruits and berries which you do not know
- do not make animals angry and be particularly careful when they have young ones with them
- learn to swim (especially if you live near water)
- encourage the local council to put up warning signs in places which are obviously dangerous
- know your neighbourhood and avoid obvious dangers
- make wells safe (children can easily fall down them)

On the road

Many deaths and serious injuries happen on the road. Children, especially, need to learn about the dangers of the road. Accidents can happen to all people who use the road. These include:

- pedestrians (people who walk on the road)
- people in cars, buses and lorries
- cyclists
- motorcyclists

Road accidents can cause death and injuries such as:

- heavy bleeding
- broken bones
- damage to main organs of the body (such as liver, lungs, brain)

Causes of road accidents

- People who drink alcohol before they drive are particularly dangerous. They do not see dangers on the road. They react slowly. They can kill themselves, other drivers, their passengers and pedestrians.

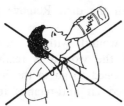

- Speed kills! Some drivers drive too fast. There are speed limits in towns and villages in most countries. They are there for good reasons. Drivers should obey them. It is always dangerous to drive fast where there are many houses, or where roads are narrow or winding.

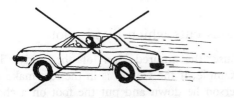

- People often drive cars and lorries which are not in good order mechanically. A car with faulty brakes will not be able to stop. Proper lights are essential.

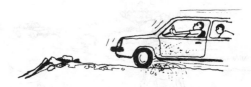

- People do not always look before they cross the road. Children, especially, may run into a road without looking.

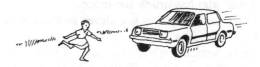

- At night, people walk along roads. Drivers sometimes do not see them, especially if they are wearing dark clothing.

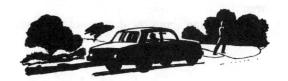

- Wet, slippery roads are dangerous.

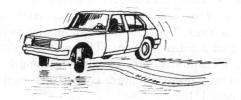

- Animals stray into the road, sometimes very suddenly. In some places, people are very angry if a driver kills their animals. Drivers thus swerve to avoid them and may crash.

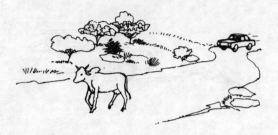

Prevention of road accidents
- Don't drink and drive. Don't ride with a driver who has drunk too much.
- Drive carefully. It is not clever to drive fast. It is dangerous.
- Drive vehicles which are safe. Check and service them often. Faulty vehicles can be killers.
- Note places where accidents often happen. Ask the local council to improve them.
- Supervise crossings near the school (Could parents help?)
- Follow road safety rules. Teach them to children.
- Teach children about the dangers of the road.

First aid

Accidents happen to everybody. They may be minor accidents such as cuts or a nose bleed, or they may be more serious such as burns or broken bones. Teachers should know what to do when an accident happens. This is called First Aid. We will give some ideas for teaching first aid to older primary children later in this chapter (see page 121).

Cuts and grazes

1 Wash your hands well. Use soap and water. Your hands have germs on them, and germs can infect the cut.

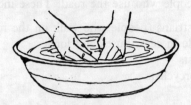

2 Wash the wound well. Use soap and water. The water should be boiled and then cooled. Germs live in unboiled water. If you boil the water you kill the germs. Rinse off the soap.

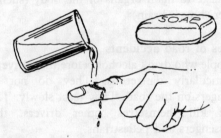

3 Clean out all the dirt. Remove small stones etc.
4 Cover the wound with a clean cloth or bandage. If the wound is really deep, the person may need to go to the health centre. He may need an anti-tetanus injection (see page 87).

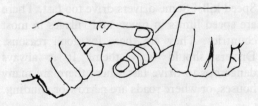

Serious cuts which bleed a lot

1 Raise the injured part of the body. For example, if the wound is in the leg, make the person lie down and put the foot on a chair.

This reduces the blood circulation to the wound, and slows down the bleeding.

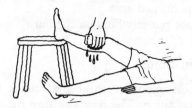

2 Press the wound with a clean cloth – or your hand if there is no cloth. Keep pressing until the bleeding stops. This may take fifteen minutes or more. Pressing causes the blood to move more slowly. It can then form a clot which is thickened and hardened blood.

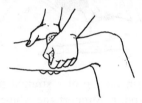

3 Tie a clean pad over the wound with a clean cloth bandage. If bleeding continues, put more pads on top. KEEP PRESSING!

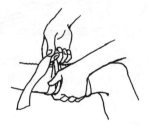

4 Take the person to the health centre as soon as possible. If people lose a lot of blood, they may die.

Nose bleed

Picking the nose, breathing hot dry, dusty air, and injury or accident to the nose can cause the nose to bleed.

1 Ask the person with the nose bleed to sit quietly. When a person sits quietly the heart beats more slowly. That causes the blood to move more slowly through the circulatory system and reduces the bleeding from the nose.

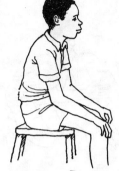

2 Put the person's head slightly forward. This will prevent him from getting dizzy.

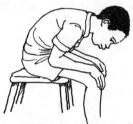

2 Put the person's head well down. This will prevent him from getting dizzy.
3 Let the person breathe through the mouth. This lets air in but does not disturb a blood clot in the nose.
4 Pinch the soft part of the nose firmly for ten minutes. This will allow a blood clot in the nose to form and helps to stop the bleeding. Tell the person to keep pinching his nose.

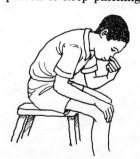

Burns and scalds

If the person's clothes are burning, put out the flames. You can stop a fire by cutting off the supply of air. So put a blanket over the person or roll him in a mat.

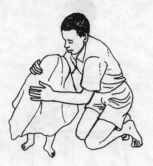

For minor burns

- **Immediately** put the burned part into cool clean water for at least ten minutes. Probably no other treatment will be necessary.

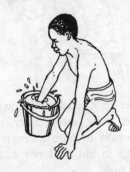

For more serious burns

- It will be necessary to take the person to the health centre or hospital
- Cover the burn with a clean dressing

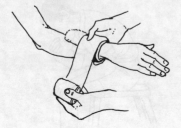

- Do not break the blisters
- Do not remove any clothing which is sticking to the burned area
- Do not put anything on the burn

Broken bones

It is most important to keep a broken bone in a fixed position. The bone can then mend itself. Here is what to do for a broken arm:

- Ask the person to lie down

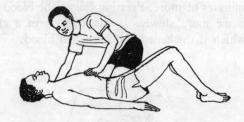

- Put the arm on top of a straight flat piece of wood or splint. Support the whole arm.

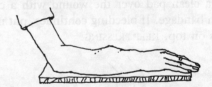

- Wrap the arm firmly to the splint with a piece of cloth. Do not wrap it too tightly as this will stop the flow of blood.

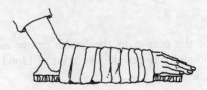

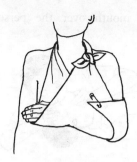

- Make a sling from another piece of cloth. The sling should hold the arm against the body.

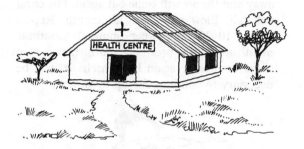

- Take the person to the health centre. The bone should be set properly so that it heals well.

How to carry a person

Two people can carry a sick person as shown here. You can make a seat with your hands.

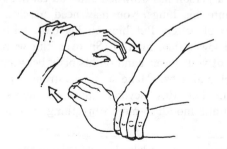

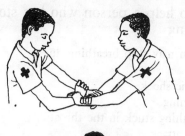

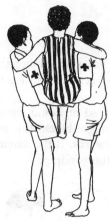

Poisoning

People, especially children, may poison themselves by drinking liquids such as kerosene or by eating tablets. Prompt action is necessary.

For poisoning from kerosene or petrol

1 DO NOT MAKE THE PERSON VOMIT. If he vomits, he may get some of the liquid in his lungs.
2 Give him some milk or water to drink. This dilutes the kerosene in the stomach.
3 Take him to the health centre immediately.

For poisoning from medicines or methylated spirits

1 MAKE THE PERSON VOMIT. You can do this by putting your finger in his throat. Or you can make him drink water with soap or salt in it.
2 He should drink as much as he can of milk, beaten eggs, or flour mixed with water.
3 Take him to the health centre immediately.

How to help a person who has stopped breathing

A person may stop breathing due to:

- electric shock
- drowning
- something stuck in the throat
- heart attack
- poisoning

A person who has stopped breathing has only four minutes to live. You must act fast!

1 Remove any food or liquid from the person's mouth. This might block their windpipe. Pull the tongue forwards. If the tongue falls back it might block the windpipe.

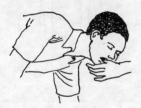

2 Put the person on his back. Tip his head back. Hold the jaw forwards. This helps to make his windpipe fully open. Air can then enter his lungs.

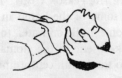

3 Pinch the person's nose, with your fingers, to close it. Otherwise when you blow into his mouth, the air will come out of his nose and not pass into his lungs.

Place your mouth over the person's open mouth.

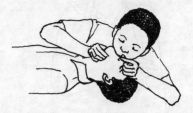

4 Blow strongly into his mouth. Watch to see that his chest rises. Now take your mouth away and the air will come out again. His chest will fall. Blow again into his mouth. Repeat about 10–20 times per minute. Continue mouth-to-mouth breathing until the person starts to breathe again by himself. It may be necessary to continue for up to an hour.

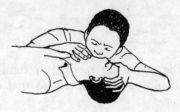

BE VERY CAREFUL WITH BABIES AND SMALL CHILDREN. DO NOT BLOW HARD OR YOU MAY BURST THEIR LUNGS. PUFF SMALL BREATHS ONLY.

If a person has drowned and you cannot blow air into his lungs, you may need to clear his lungs of water. Put him on his back with his head lower than his feet. Sit over him with the heel of your lower hand on his belly between his navel and ribs. Make a quick strong upward push. Do this several times if necessary. Continue mouth-to-mouth breathing at once.

The first aid which has been described above covers only the most common accidents. Try to do a proper first aid course. You should, for example, know about treatment for shock or snake bite and how to deal with serious wounds.

Some Teaching Suggestions

Finding out about accidents

The subject of safety may not be immediately interesting to children. You can make it more interesting by showing them that it is **relevant** to their lives. Accidents happen to every one. In some accidents, people are killed or injured seriously. Often accidents can be prevented. Encourage children to find out about accidents. They could find about national accidents and local accidents:

- From the newspaper. Either you or the children could cut out stories about accidents from a newspaper. Make a class scrapbook about them. Put the scrapbook on the wall.
- From the radio news. Either at school or at home, ask the children to listen to the news on the radio. What accidents are reported?
- From their own reports. What accidents have happened at home? At school? On the way to school? They could keep a record of accidents either in exercise books, or on a chart on the wall.

	Week 1	Week 2	Week 3
at school	II	I	
at home	IIII	┼┼┼I	
in the neighbourhood	┼┼┼	II	
on the road	I	III	

For any accident, children could discuss and write about it. You could ask these questions to help them think about it:

- who had the accident?
- where did it happen?
- when did it happen?
- what injuries were caused?
- what caused the accident?
- what action did people take after the accident?
- how could it have been prevented?

Teaching ideas

Spot the hazard

Get the children to look around the classroom and list anything which is not safe.

Ask the children:

- what accidents might happen in the classroom?
- what injuries might result?
- how can we make our classroom a safer place?

Let them do a similar activity for other areas of the school such as the playground or other classrooms.

Picture stories

Put large pictures, like those shown here, on the wall.

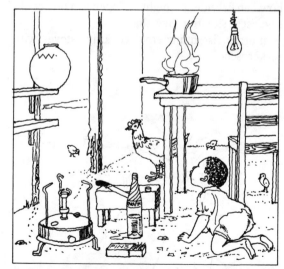

What could cause accidents in the picture shown here and over the page? Get children to list possible causes of accidents.

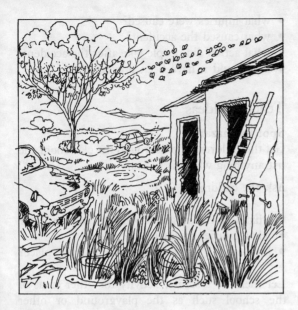

- visitor comes to house and mother goes to the door
- small child, who is left by himself, picks up the kerosene bottle and drinks from it

You could organise poster competitions. Children could draw posters warning about hazards at home or in the neighbourhood. You could hold a competition to see who can draw the best ones. Some examples are illustrated below.

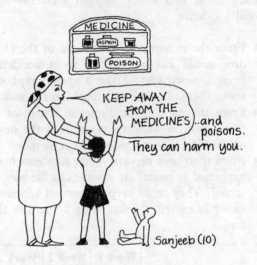

MEDICINE

ASPIRIN

POISON

KEEP AWAY FROM THE MEDICINES ...and poisons. They can harm you.

Sanjeeb (10)

Can the children draw their own picture stories to show hazards at home or at school? Put the good ones on the wall. Let other children discuss them. Can they make a series of drawings to show how an accident might happen? You could suggest a situation like this:

- mother is filling the cooking stove with kerosene

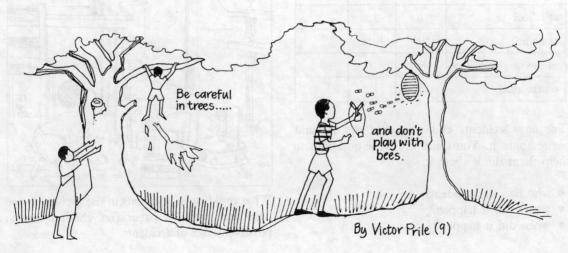

Be careful in trees.....

and don't play with bees.

By Victor Prile (9)

Use the school rules

Show children the school rules. Ask them which ones are there to prevent accidents. When they have had a chance to observe possible hazards in the playground and classroom, ask them to make a set of school rules for themselves. Let the children work in groups for this activity so that they can share their ideas. The whole class might then put the good rules together and make a set of rules for the school. You could use this as an opportunity to discuss school rules generally.

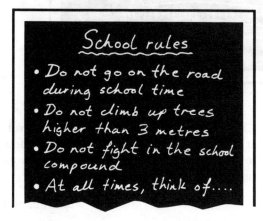

Stories and plays

Make up stories about common accidents which happen in the school, home or neighbourhood. You could use some of the ideas from this chapter, for example:

- a baby is scalded
- a child cuts herself on a knife
- a boy falls out of a tree
- a girl often plays with a ball near to the road
- a baby eats a bottle of aspirin pills

Let the children discuss the story. Can they say how the accident could have been prevented? Can they suggest what first aid should be given in each case.

Can the children make up their own stories? If they are suitable, encourage them to tell the stories to their younger brothers and sisters at home.

Let the children make up plays about accidents. Let them work out an outline first.

Here is one idea for a typical plot:

- Child is knocked down by a car at a dangerous corner. Policemen are called. Angry crowd scene. Child is taken to hospital. Parents meet to decide what action to take. A complaint is sent to the Council. The Council hears evidence about the dangerous corner.

Children could act out different plays in groups. The other children in the class could try to decide:

- what caused the accident?
- how could it have been prevented?
- who behaved well in the play?
- who behaved badly?

Always have a discussion after each play. The children should think about the important messages which the play contains.

Make maps

On a large piece of paper, or the blackboard, draw a map of the village or neighbourhood. Make the map as simple as possible. Draw the main roads and footpaths. Let the children suggest where to put other landmarks such as the school, the railway, the health clinic, the market, the mosque or church, shops, their own houses. Now they can suggest places where accidents have happened or are likely to happen. You could mark these places with a special symbol. The illustration on page 118 shows what such a map might look like.

The children could also make a model of the village or neighbourhood. They could make models of houses and other buildings and put them in the correct places on the model.

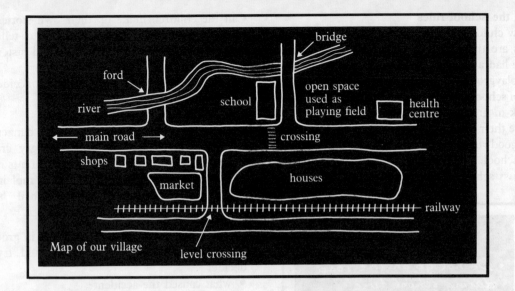

Map of our village

They could mark places where accidents have happened by small flags. They could make the flag from a stick and piece of paper.

Discuss these maps or models with the children. There are more ideas about making maps in chapter 11.

Preventing accidents around the school

Children can help to keep the school compound safe and clean. You could organise them to clear away rubbish, or to cut long grass. Groups of children could be responsible for different parts of the compound. Perhaps there could be a competition between the groups. (See chapter 10.)

Safety on the road

Teach the children how to behave on the road. If possible, obtain a copy of the Highway Code. Here are some important rules which children should learn:

- Choose a safe place when crossing the road. It is dangerous to cross near a corner or near to the top of a hill. It is dangerous to cross near to a parked vehicle.

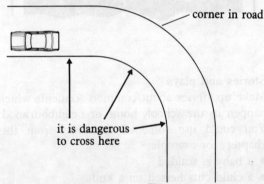

Discuss with children why these places are dangerous. If they must cross near to a parked vehicle, they should come to the outside corner of the vehicle first. Then they can see the road clearly before they cross. (See diagram on page 119.)

- If there is a crossing for pedestrians, use it.
- Look both ways before crossing. Cross only if the road is clear.

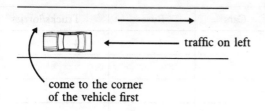

traffic on left

come to the corner of the vehicle first

- Walk across the road. Do not run.
- If there is no pavement (sidewalk), walk along the side of the road which faces the traffic. (For countries which drive on the left, this means the right side of the road. For countries which drive on the right, this means the left side of the road.)

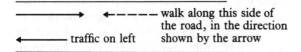

traffic on left — walk along this side of the road, in the direction shown by the arrow

- Wear light-coloured clothes at night.

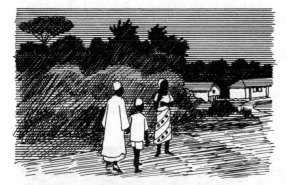

- On the road, look after younger children.

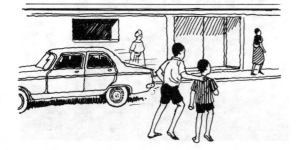

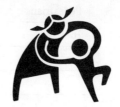

Draw a road safety map on the board or on a large piece of paper. (It could be like the one suggested on page 121 for accidents.) Show on the map the main paths or roads which children use when coming to school. Ask them:
- where do they cross the road?
- where have accidents happened?
- which places on the roads need special care?

Mark these places on the map and discuss them with the children.

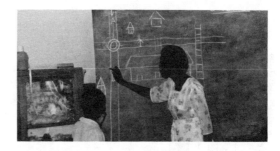

Do a traffic survey. Use the information from the road safety map above to choose a place to do the survey. Decide with the children what information to collect. Ask them:
- Which vehicles will they count?
- When will they watch? Will they watch throughout the day?
- Will they watch at the same time for an hour every day of the week?

(You will need to fit in the survey to suit your timetable.)
Make sure that the children will behave sensibly, especially if they are near to a dangerous road.

119

	Pedestrians	Bikes	Cars	Buses	Trucks/lorries
0800–0900	16	7	5	3	4
0900–1000					
1000–1100					
1100–1200					
1200–1300					
1300–1400					
1400–1500					
TOTAL	150				

Let us suppose that they do a survey throughout one day. They might record the information in a table like the one shown above.

They could then transfer this information to bar graphs like these:

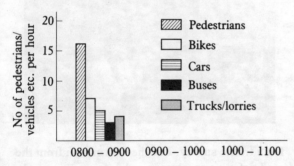

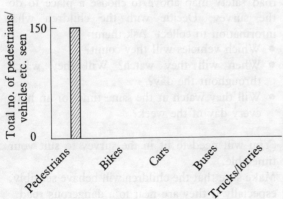

Discuss with the children the information which the bar graph and table shows. Encourage them to look out for dangerous behaviour by drivers or pedestrians while they do the survey. Let them tell the rest of the class about it.

Ask children to observe people's behaviour on the road as they come to school. For example, do they use crossings? Are people who get off the bus careful about crossing the road? What dangerous incidents did they observe?

Use the school compound to teach children about road safety. Draw 'roadways' on the ground. Let children practise crossing the road.

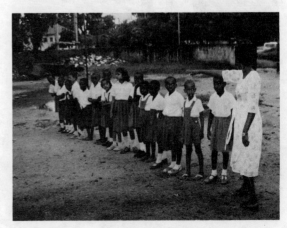

Make it more interesting by creating some dangerous situations. You could put a bend in the road and let some children be stationary vehicles. The other children could then show how they would cross. Teach them the danger of running into the road without looking. Let them run up to the side of an imaginary road and then try to stop. If they try to stop only at the side of the road, they will find that they actually stop moving in the middle of the road.

Draw some road situations on the board. Get children to say where accidents might happen. Make the drawing very simple like this:

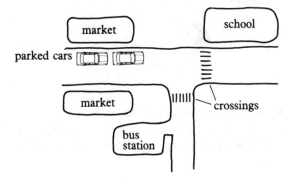

Make up a song about road safety or get the children to suggest one. Here is an example (with the music shown):

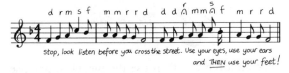

stop, look listen before you cross the street. Use your eyes, use your ears and THEN use your feet!

Children could teach the song to their younger brothers and sisters.

Teaching first aid

Use the suggestions below together with the background knowledge about first aid on pages 110 to 114.

Cuts and bleeding
- Draw a cut on the child's skin. Ask the children to make a list of what they will need to treat it. Let them say or write down what they would do.
- Show them how to control serious bleeding from a wound in the leg or arm. Then let them practise on each other.
- Show them what to do for a nose bleed. Then let them practise on each other.

Injured arms and legs
Show the children what to do if someone has a broken arm (page 112). Show them how to put on a splint and sling. Let them practise on each other in small groups. You will need the following materials:
- bamboo canes or straight wood sticks for splints
- some triangular bandages (you could use instead of these, scarves or squares of cloth folded in half)

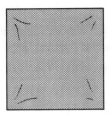 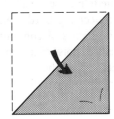

- clean strips of cloth for bandages

Let them also practise how to carry an injured person (page 113).

Burns and scalds
Show children that air is needed for burning. Place a jar over a lighted candle like this:

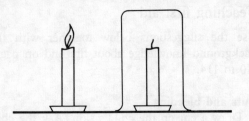

The candle goes out because it does not have enough air (strictly speaking it uses a proportion of the oxygen in the air).

The same principle is used if a person is on fire. Quickly wrap him in a blanket to keep away the air. Let the children try this. One child pretends that his clothes are burning. The other children then throw a blanket over him and wrap it around him. They could try this in small groups.

Let them also practise what to do if a person is scalded. The injured part of the body should be put into clean cold water as soon as possible (see page 112). If possible, have a bucket of water available.

Poisoning

- Teach the children about poisoning from kerosene or petrol or from taking too much medicine (see page 113).
- Collect old bottles and tins. Label them with the names of common substances which often cause poisoning (kerosene, petrol, aspirins, etc.). Get the children to say what the treatment is for each.

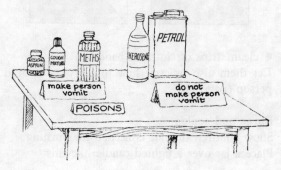

A person who has stopped breathing

Teach children how to deal with someone who has stopped breathing (perhaps from drowning or electric shock). Show them how to do mouth-to-mouth breathing on each other. If they are embarrassed about this then make a model according to the following instructions:

- get a plastic bottle

- cut a hole for the mouth and two holes for the nostrils

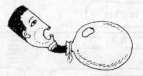

- paint the bottle to look like a head
- connect it to a balloon or polythene bag with a tube (such as an inner tube from a bicycle tyre)

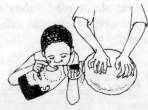

The children can then use the model to practise mouth-to-mouth breathing.

First aid plays

Children could work in groups to make a drama about an accident and then give first aid to the person. The other children could try to judge whether they give the correct first aid to their patient.

Chapter Seven

Deadly decisions

Useful Background Knowledge

Habits and decisions

This chapter is about:

- smoking
- drinking alcohol
- taking drugs

You may wonder why we include a chapter like this in a book for primary school teachers. The reason is that attitudes form very early in the lives of children. By the end of primary school, they may have formed very clear attitudes about smoking, drinking alcohol, and taking drugs. Moreover, for many children in developing countries, primary school may be the only formal educational institution that they attend. The primary school thus has a responsibility to ensure that children are aware of the dangers to health which may be caused by these activities.

A **habit** is something which we do regularly. Sometimes a habit becomes so much a part of us that we do it without thinking. We often learn a habit from our friends or from other people. Habits are formed as a result of decisions which we take. We can **decide** about smoking, drinking alcohol and taking drugs. The decisions which we make may be literally **deadly** in their consequences, as you will read in the rest of this chapter.

However, remember that these problems are not serious everywhere. Some religions forbid alcohol and smoking. In many places, fortunately, abuse (or wrong use) of drugs is not a problem. As you read this chapter, bear in mind the social situation where you live. Adjust your teaching accordingly. Consult with other teachers and the head-teacher to decide what you will teach and how you will teach it.

Smoking

The effects of smoking on the body

Look again at page 38 where the breathing system is explained. When we breathe in, air passes through the nose and mouth, into the windpipe, and then into the tiny air sacs in the lungs. If a person smokes, this whole delicate system is damaged, for tobacco contains three harmful substances:

- **nicotine**, which increases the rate at which the heart beats
- **tar**, which lines the tubes which lead into the lungs
- **carbon monoxide**, which affects the ability of the blood to carry oxygen.

When a person smokes, these substances and pieces of burned tobacco pass into the tubes and lungs. They irritate the delicate linings. Normally, the windpipe is lined by tiny hairs (or **cilia**) which move backward and forwards. Over the cilia is a sticky liquid which is called **mucus**. The mucus traps tiny pieces of dust and

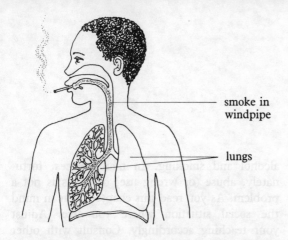

smoke in
windpipe

lungs

dirt which are in the air. The cilia move the
mucus upwards at the rate of about $1\frac{1}{2}$ cm every
minute. Eventually the mucus reaches the throat
where we swallow it (or sometimes spit it out).

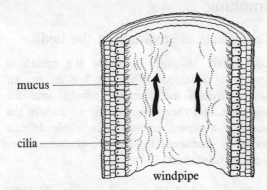

mucus

cilia

windpipe

highly magnified

If smoke passes into the air tubes, it will cause
the cilia to slow down their movement and eventually stop. The mucus no longer passes upwards
and therefore drops down into the air sacs. The
person then has to cough to get rid of it. A
person who smokes a lot often has a bad cough.
He may eventually get a disease called **bronchitis**. This is when the tubes leading to the
lungs become inflamed. He has to cough
frequently to remove the mucus which gathers
in the lungs.

124

Smoking also affects other parts of the body.
Smoking just one cigarette causes:

- the skin temperature to drop
- the heart to beat faster
- the blood pressure to rise

Smoking and health

SMOKING IS DANGEROUS!

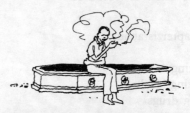

You will understand from the above that
smoking can have a most serious effect upon a
person's health. Consider the facts:

- If you smoke for many years, you are likely
  to become very ill. You can shorten your life
  by 10–15 years.

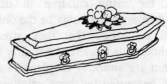

- On average, a smoker shortens his life by
  about $5\frac{1}{2}$ minutes for each cigarette which he
  smokes.

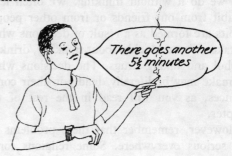

There goes another
$5\frac{1}{2}$ minutes

- If children begin to smoke, they are affected as much as adults. They get more coughs, colds, and shortness of breath.

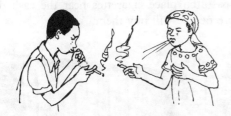

- Smoking damages the sense of taste. The hot smoke and other chemicals in smoke affect the taste buds. The sense of smell is also affected.

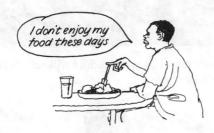

- Smoking makes teeth go yellow. Clothes, hair, and breath smell of smoke and ash.

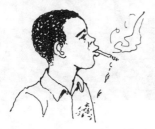

- People who smoke are more likely to suffer from heart disease. Smoking often makes stomach ulcers worse and can cause them.

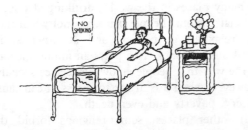

- Worst of all, people who smoke are much more likely to get cancer, especially lung cancer. Cancer is an uncontrolled growth of the cells. Normally, cells die and are replaced naturally. However, when a person has cancer the cells grow out of control to form lumps. The lining of the lungs is affected and eventually a cancerous growth will form.

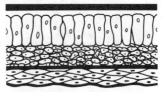

normal lining of the lung

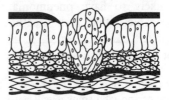

lining of lung showing cancerous growth

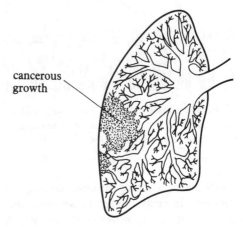

cancerous growth

section through a lung

125

- If a pregnant woman smokes, she affects the growth of her baby. Nicotine and carbon monoxide pass via the mother's blood across the placenta to the baby's blood. The baby is likely to be smaller, more underdeveloped, and less resistant to disease.

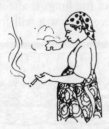

- In families where parents smoke, children are more likely to have pneumonia and other diseases which affect their breathing.

Smoking is very risky. A smoker has up to twenty-five times the risk of getting lung cancer compared with a non-smoker. This is not to say that every person who smokes will get lung cancer. But nine out of every ten people with lung cancer are smokers.

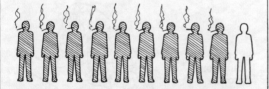

Smoking also causes cancer of the mouth and throat. Here, the risk for a smoker is ten times the risk for a non-smoker.

Remember, also, some of the other consequences of smoking. It costs money to smoke. Money which is spent on cigarettes is money which is not spent on more useful things (such as on food and clothing for the family).

A person who is sick from an illness caused by smoking takes up the health resources of a country. The time and attention of health workers, doctors, and nurses, is taken up by people who need not be ill.

Advertisers put pressure on people to smoke. Shops often place cigarettes near the cash desk where people will buy them.

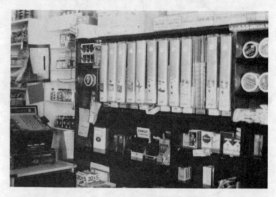

In many places, street vendors will sell cigarettes in twos or threes.

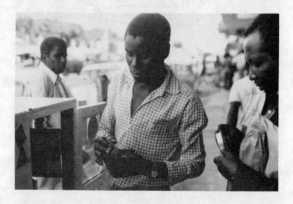

Drinking alcohol

In many places in the world, drinking alcohol is a social custom. People drink alcohol when they are relaxing, at parties, and at other social occasions. Alcohol often plays an important part in the way that people enjoy themselves socially. However, when it is drunk to excess, it can cause misery, poverty and even death.

In other places, some religions forbid the

drinking of alcohol. Thus the problems which may arise when people drink too much alcohol are not serious everywhere.

Below are some of the facts about alcohol, its effects on the body, and on people's health.

The effects of drinking alcohol on the body

Different drinks contain different amounts of alcohol. Beer contains approximately 5%–8% alcohol, wine about 10% alcohol, and spirits (such as whisky) 40% alcohol.

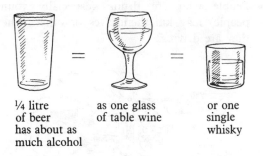

¼ litre of beer has about as much alcohol   as one glass of table wine   or one single whisky

When a person drinks alcohol, it passes into his stomach. From there, it passes into the blood in which it is carried to the brain. This takes between 5–10 minutes.

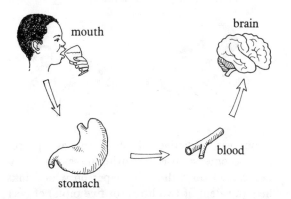

The amount of alcohol in the blood depends on a number of factors:

- the amount of alcohol drunk
- whether the person's stomach is full or not
- how heavy the person is

The amount of alcohol in the blood rises for a while after the person stops drinking. It then falls as the liver breaks the alcohol down into simpler substances. The graph shows how the amount of alcohol varies in the blood of a man who drinks a litre (1¾pints) of beer.

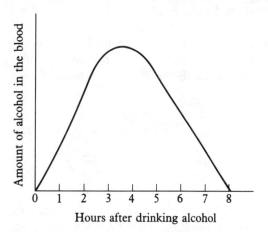

The brain controls the whole nervous system of the body. It controls the way in which we think and determines how we behave. Alcohol affects the brain temporarily. It affects the way we see and feel things.

People sometimes think that alcohol is a stimulant. In fact, the opposite is true. It actually slows down the body's responses. The result is that a person cannot judge situations properly. This is particularly important if he then drives a car or motor cycle. His reactions will be slow and his judgement of traffic situations will be poor. He is much more likely to have a crash.

In many countries of the world, there are laws about drinking alcohol and driving. Drivers who have a certain amount of alcohol in their blood may be fined, lose their licence, or even sent to prison. What do **you** think about laws like this?

Alcohol affects people's behaviour. Some people laugh more. Others become sleepy or aggressive. Young people, particularly, may lose their self-control and do silly or violent things.

Alcohol and health

In small quantities, alcohol does no harm to a person's health. However, when people begin to drink a lot they run a serious risk to their physical health and social well-being. These are likely to be the results:

- Physically, they are more likely to suffer from liver and heart disease, pneumonia, ulcers, and cancer of the digestive system.

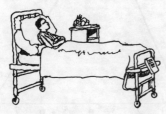

- Mentally, they become depressed when they are not drinking. They lose their self-respect.

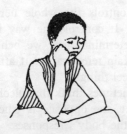

- At work, they have problems with their jobs, and in their relationships with other people.

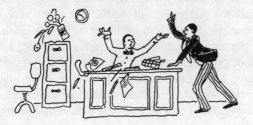

- It is probably at home that the situation becomes worst of all. A drunken man may hit his wife and children. A drunken woman may abuse her husband and children. Families may split up.

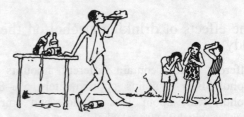

- People who are drunk (especially young people) may kill themselves or others when they are driving.

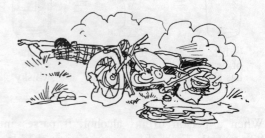

- People who drink heavily waste a lot of money. Money is spent on alcohol rather than on healthy food for the family.

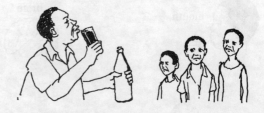

Alcohol is addictive. That is to say, people may become so used to drinking alcohol that they cannot do without it. A person who drinks the equivalent of two litres (or five pints) of beer a day is in danger of becoming an alcoholic. An alcoholic has to drink alcohol in order to feel normal.

Drugs

When we speak of drugs, we tend to think of **illegal** drugs such as marijuana or cocaine. However, we have seen that alcohol is a kind of drug. Medicines which we take when we are ill are also drugs. An anaesthetic which is used to make a person unconscious during an operation is a drug.

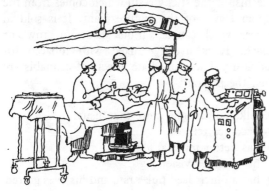

There are some drugs which can be given only by a health worker or doctor. There are others which we can buy across the counter in a chemist's shop. There are still others which are illegal. It is important to be clear that the terms **drug** and **drug abuse** are not confined only to the illegal drugs.

The effect of drugs on the body

Drugs may be taken by mouth, they may be breathed in, or they may be injected. The drug passes into the blood which carries it around the

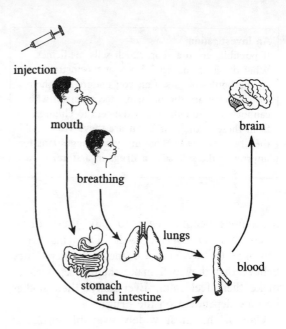

body. Many drugs affect the brain. The brain, via the nervous system, controls the rest of the body.

When a person takes a drug regularly, his body begins to get used to it. Without the drug, the person's body does not feel normal so he has to take more of it. He is then **dependent** on the drug. He has an intense desire for it. It is then very difficult for him to give up the drug.

The kinds of drugs

As we have seen, alcohol and tobacco are two drugs which people often use. Modern medicine has produced a great variety of different drugs (or medicines) which are used to treat illnesses. These drugs bring great benefit. They can prevent pain and heal sickness.

Yet sometimes these drugs are abused (wrongly used). They are often freely available in shops and stores so that people can buy them easily.

Sometimes people begin to buy these drugs when they do not feel well. They may then continue to buy and use them. Perhaps they believe that they will make them sleep well or make them feel calm. Eventually, their bodies become dependent on the drugs.

One of the most widely available drugs is **aspirin** which helps to kill pain. Sometimes, people can become dependent on it, taking aspirin continuously. If it is taken often, it can cause bleeding of the stomach.

Sedatives and stimulants

Sedatives make people feel drowsy or sleepy. They calm the activity of the brain. Stimulants (sometimes called 'pep' pills) make them feel lively. They speed up the activity of the brain. However, when their effect wears off, the person often feels tired and exhausted.

Hallucinogens

Other kinds of drug which cause people to see and feel things in a very strange way are called **hallucinogens**. They are dangerous because they change the way in which a person sees the world around him. They sometimes lead him to think that he can do things of which he is really incapable. They will affect his judgement and physical skills. An example is the drug called 'LSD'. It is also known as 'acid' and is used in the form of pills.

These drugs are illegal because:

- they seriously affect people's behaviour
- they are harmful to the user and to the people around him.

Thus a person who uses them will not only damage his health. He is also likely to be arrested if he is caught using them, or if he sells or gives them to anyone else.

Marijuana and hashish

These dangerous drugs come from the hemp (or cannabis) plant. They are two of the most common illegal drugs. They are usually smoked in hand-rolled cigarettes or specially made pipes. Marijuana, which is the dried leaves of the plant, is greyish or greenish brown and looks like tea. Hashish is the sticky resin which comes from the upper leaves of the mature plant. It is sold in pieces which can be various shades of brown or black. It is usually mixed with tobacco for smoking. The immediate effects of cannabis are that the person:

- talks and laughs more than usual
- becomes relaxed
- has better musical ability
- has sharper vision
- has an increased pulse rate and his eyes go red
- later becomes quiet and sleepy

Some of these effects may seem attractive to you. That is why people start the habit. But once they start, it is very difficult to stop. The body begins to need more and more because it gets used to having it. Then the user begins to notice other effects. He may get restless, tired, or confused, and be unable to remember things. This is especially common in teenagers and young adults.

Heavy use of cannabis is dangerous to health. The tar content of cannabis smoke is at least 50% higher than that of tobacco. Heavy users of cannabis are much more likely to get chronic bronchitis, lung cancer, and other lung diseases.

Why do people smoke, drink, and take drugs?

In this chapter, we have explained that:

- smoking and taking illegal drugs is never good for health
- drinking alcohol to excess is likely to be dangerous to health

Why then do people smoke, drink to excess and use illegal drugs? You may like to discuss this question among yourselves, with other students or your tutor. Some aspects which you may like to consider are the following:

- Do people really enjoy doing these things?
- Do they like doing it the first time? If not, why do they persist? Is it to prove to themselves and others that they are really grown up? How in your society do people mark the change from childhood to adulthood? Are traditional customs fading?
- Do people do these things to forget their problems? To escape temporarily from personal tragedy, poverty, or tiredness of life?
- Do they want to impress other people? Do they want to do what their friends do, to be 'one of the crowd'? Do they want to seem important?
- Have they been persuaded by advertisements?

When you consider these questions, think about children of primary age. Remember that some of them will be approaching the time when they have to make **decisions** about these habits. Will they start to smoke when they are offered a cigarette? Do they have enough information about the effects of smoking on health?

The role of advertisements

An advertisement tries to persuade people to buy certain products. The advertisement illustrated here is advertising cigarettes. It is trying to persuade people that successful sportsmen smoke their brand of cigarette. Of course, the truth is that a sportsman will be less good if he smokes.

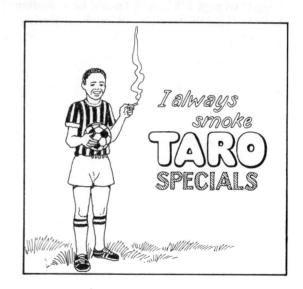

Advertisers of cigarettes often try to link the idea of **health** to the product which they are selling. This is dishonest for the link between smoking and **ill health** is proved beyond reasonable doubt. Tobacco companies often sponsor sports events. Look, for example, at the poster illustrated here, which is advertising a sporting event (it was, in fact, placed at the entrance to a primary school!).

Look at advertisements for drinks and medicines. How do the advertisers try to sell these products? What kind of people appear in them? What is the hidden message which they carry? The techniques of the advertisers are clever and subtle. They use attractive or famous people to persuade you to buy particular products. We suggest on page 138 how you might help children to understand the pressures which the advertisers try to exert.

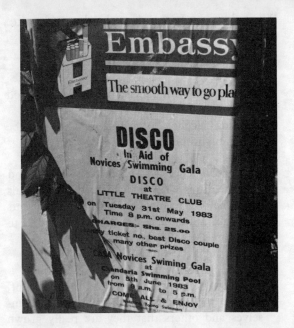

Some Teaching Suggestions

Planning the work

It is particularly important to plan this work carefully. Decide first whether it is necessary to cover all three areas of smoking, drinking alcohol and drug abuse. Which, if any, are problems in your community or for your children? It may be, for example, that many children are likely to become smokers, but that drinking alcohol to excess and drug abuse are not problems. In any case, remember that teaching about these subjects will be much more relevant at the top end of the primary school. It is then that children will be making decisions which determine their future response to these habits.

It is important that children should know the facts about the effects of these substances on their health. But this is not enough. Children need to examine the pressures which may force them towards taking up the habits discussed in this chapter.

Set an example

Teaching by example is always powerful. If you yourself smoke or drink to excess, children will find it hard to believe you. They will copy you as an adult. If you do smoke, try to give it up. If you cannot give it up, try not to smoke at school or where the children can see you.

Facts, debates, posters

Read the first section of this chapter 'Useful Background Knowledge'. Make sure that children are at least aware of the facts about smoking, alcohol and drug abuse. Read the relevant section of chapter 2 about the breathing and circulatory systems of the body.

- A good way to begin might be by a **word association game**. For instance, you could play the game with smoking as the topic.

The teacher calls out a leading word such as 'lung cancer'. A child now calls out a word which he associates with this such as 'illness,' 'hospital' or 'cigarettes'. Other children then call out other words which they associate with the leading word. Encourage them to suggest words related to smoking. Pause from time to time to discuss the associations which children make. Encourage the positive as well as negative ideas. For example, 'lung cancer' might be followed by 'give up smoking'.

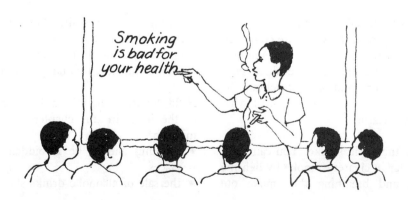

- Make up a **true/false quiz** for the children. Here are some ideas:

1 It is estimated that every cigarette which you smoke shortens your life by one minute	**T/F**
2 The smoke which a smoker breathes out can harm other people	**T/F**
3 If a person who smokes ten cigarettes a day stops smoking, he can save about – (choose a suitable amount of money)	**T/F**
4 If a person smokes, he will definitely get lung cancer	**T/F**
5 Smoking by a pregnant mother can damage the health of her unborn baby	**T/F**
6 Alcohol is a stimulant	**T/F**
7 Anyone who drinks alcohol will become an alcoholic	**T/F**
8 A small amount of alcohol improves your performance in certain physical activities like driving	**T/F**
9 It is quite safe to smoke marijuana	**T/F**
10 People can become dependent on drugs like aspirin	**T/F**

Answers

1 **False**   It is estimated that the average figure is $5\frac{1}{2}$ minutes for each cigarette smoked

2 **True**   A study was carried out over a period of fourteen years in Japan. It tried to discover what happened to non-smoking women who were married to smokers. The women were twice as likely to die as women who were married to non-smokers.

3 **False**   Insert a suitable figure in your own currency (less than might be expected)

4 **False**   A smoker will not definitely get lung cancer. However, it has been shown statistically that he is up to twenty five times more likely to get it than a non-smoker.

5 **True**   The substances in smoke pass into the mother's blood. From there, they can reach the unborn baby.

6 **False**   Alcohol slows down the activity of the brain

7 **False**   Alcohol in small amounts does no harm. The danger is that people begin to drink too much alcohol and become dependent on it.

8 **False**   Even a small amount of alcohol affects the way in which a person drives

9 **False**   Marijuana is a dangerous drug which can affect people's health

10 **True**   It is possible for people to abuse even common drugs which are quite safe when used sensibly

Make up similar true/false statements of your own. Base them on the facts which are contained earlier in this chapter rather than on opinions. Perhaps you could use the quiz to evaluate children's learning before and after teaching the topic. This will give you an indication of what the children have learnt.

- Demonstrate the tar in smoke. You can show children the tar in cigarette smoke by lighting a cigarette, and breathing the smoke out through a clean white cloth (like a handkerchief). A stain will appear on it. This stain is tar. Point out to the children that when a smoker inhales, this tar goes into his lungs.

Hold debates. Organise a debate based on some of the ideas in this chapter. Possible motions might be:
- smoking should be forbidden in all public places
- the sale of alcoholic drinks should be banned

- the government should double the price of cigarettes

Let two children speak for two minutes for and against the motion. Encourage them to work out carefully what they will say beforehand. Let other children also speak. It is probably best if you, the teacher, act as chairman. Listen to the points which they make. Summarise what they say. Help them to distinguish valid points.

Make posters about smoking, drinking alcohol, and (if relevant) drug abuse. Teach children the principles of good posters:
- They should be 'eye catching' (attractive)
- They are advertisements for good health (you want people to notice and read them)
- A good poster has a good caption. For example:
  'Smoking can kill you'
  'Drink less, eat more'
  'When you get the habit, the habit gets you'
  'Drink . . . drive . . . dead'
  Can the children think of their own captions? Use the information which the children have collected about the costs of smoking and drinking. Can they make posters for people who cannot read? When you have some good posters from the class, visit the health centre or hospital. Ask them if they would like to display the posters which the children have made.

Learning to say 'no'

Introduce role-play on 'learning to say no'. Many people who smoke get the habit when they are children. The most powerful pressure to smoke often comes from friends. Teachers can help children to be aware of this pressure. They can help them to say 'no'. Role-plays can be effective. Here is an idea for a situation which children could act:

- Five children arrange to meet at their favourite meeting place. One of them produces some cigarettes and offers them to the others. One of them says 'No, thank you. I don't smoke'. The others ask 'Why not?' What does he say? The others try to persuade him. How does he deal with this pressure?

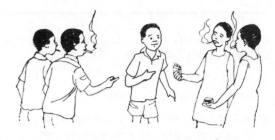

Discuss with the class how the person who did not wish to smoke might react. What things might he do and say? Here are some suggestions:

- walk away
- argue with the others
- suggest something else to do
- ask the others why they smoke
- point out that smoking wastes money
- tell the others what a filthy habit it is
- make excuses
- find new friends!
- tell them how it will damage their health

Breaking the habit

Many people decide not to smoke. But many others do. Later in their lives, smokers may want to stop but find it very hard to give up the habit.

Let children work in pairs to list:
- the benefits of being a non-smoker
- what you can do to help stop smoking

Combine the lists to make a class list. Write the ideas on a big sheet of paper:

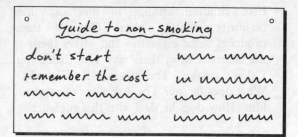

Guide to non-smoking

don't start

remember the cost

Put up the chart in the classroom or use it at a school health convention. (See page 199)

What is the cost of smoking?

- Ask children to find out the cost of a packet of cigarettes. From this they can calculate how much one costs. They could ask an adult smoker how many he smokes in one day, and from this calculate how many he smokes in a week. How much does it cost him each week? Collect as much information as possible from the class. Can they calculate from this information how much an average smoker spends on cigarettes each week? Can they suggest what else he could buy for this amount of money? (Food, clothes, a bicycle for example.)

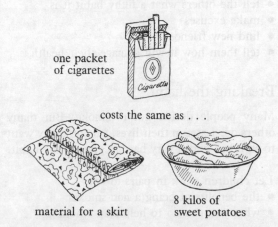

one packet
of cigarettes

costs the same as . . .

material for a skirt

8 kilos of
sweet potatoes

- Can they estimate how many people in the community smoke? What is the total amount

of money spent on cigarettes each week (using the average which they have calculated above)? What is the total cost in a year? What could the community do with this amount of money?

Is tobacco grown locally? Could the children find out about this? How much do farmers sell the crop for? Would they get more money if they grew other crops?

What is the cost of drinking alcohol?

- Can children find out what local alcoholic drinks cost? How much does a bottle or can of beer cost for instance? How much does it cost in one week if a person drinks a bottle of beer a day? What could he buy with this amount of money?

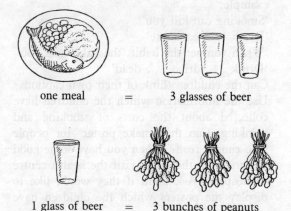

one meal = 3 glasses of beer

1 glass of beer = 3 bunches of peanuts

Both for smoking and drinking alcohol, help children to understand how much money may be wasted on them. Help them to realise that once people have the habit, it is difficult to get rid of it. They have to spend money to keep the habit going.

Finding out about drugs

Visit the local store with the children. (You may have to make the visit with only a few children at a time.) They could observe:

- which drugs are on sale
- what they cost
- where they are kept in the shop
- whether children can reach them easily

When they return to the classroom, they could work together to make a list of the drugs which were on sale.

A typical store might, for example, sell the following:

> aspirin
> paracetamol
> gripe water
> throat tablets
> antiseptic cream

Discuss with the children where the drugs were kept. Was it the best place? What are the dangers in selling these drugs?

- Ask children to make a list of the drugs which they can find at home. Which drugs were bought in a store? Which drugs did a health worker or doctor give to someone in the family? Where in the home are the drugs kept? Can all members of the family read the instructions?

They could record their findings like this:

DRUG	WHERE BOUGHT	WHERE KEPT	WHO CANNOT READ?
Aspirin Cough mixture	Store Health worker	Bedroom (floor) kitchen cupboard	Baby Sam Mother

Discuss the children's findings with them. Do they recognise the dangers – and the benefits – of these drugs?

- Try to get some labels of common drugs which are sold in a store. These could be from old jars or bottles. A store keeper might be able to give you some. Make a visual aid for the children. This should show them what they can learn from the label. Stick the label on to a large sheet of paper.

- Can the children themselves design labels for common medicines? Can they suggest ideas to help people who may not be able to read?

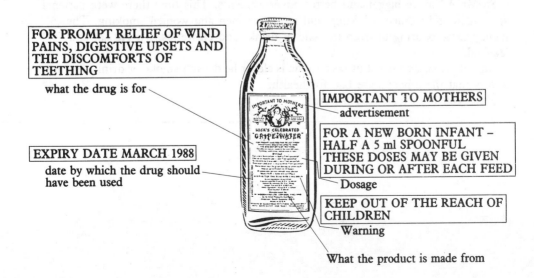

FOR PROMPT RELIEF OF WIND PAINS, DIGESTIVE UPSETS AND THE DISCOMFORTS OF TEETHING
what the drug is for

EXPIRY DATE MARCH 1988
date by which the drug should have been used

IMPORTANT TO MOTHERS
advertisement

FOR A NEW BORN INFANT – HALF A 5 ml SPOONFUL THESE DOSES MAY BE GIVEN DURING OR AFTER EACH FEED
Dosage

KEEP OUT OF THE REACH OF CHILDREN
Warning

What the product is made from

Understanding advertisements

Tell the children a story about the people who make advertisements for cigarettes and alcohol. Here is a suggestion for one:

Get the children to draw a picture of the story. Discuss it with them. Ask them questions about it, such as:

- why does Mr Ad make advertisements?
- why does he change them from time to time?
- who pays Mr Ad in real life?

Mr Ad is a nasty man. He tries to force people into bad habits. He is behind the poster which says 'Drink beer', and the advertisement which says 'Smoke cigarettes'.

Mr Ad has been in business for a long time. He is very clever. For every time that someone buys a bottle of beer, or a packet of cigarettes, he gets richer and richer.

But a few years ago, Mr Ad found that he was not getting as much money as before. He began to realise that health workers, teachers, doctors and nurses were telling people not to smoke and drink. People began to understand how bad these things were for their health.

'I'll show them!' he said, 'I'll prove how weak these people really are!' So he put his advertisements on the radio and television. He drew bigger and better pictures in the newspaper. Some of these were in colour in glossy magazines. This brought in more money, but not as much as he had hoped, for he is very greedy for money. He knows that there are more well-educated young people leaving school. He knows that they can read well, and he knows that they would like to be smart in some way.

'They will soon forget their health lessons' he thought, 'when they see smart people drinking and smoking'.

So Mr Ad made bigger and better advertisements. This time there were national sportsmen and women drinking, and attractive men and women smoking. The money came pouring in from the sale of drinks and cigarettes. Mr Ad sat and laughed.

Mr Ad is a nasty man. But because he is clever he doesn't smoke or drink, for he knows that these habits are bad for health.

Have **you** been fooled by Mr Ad?

Collect advertisements for cigarettes, alcoholic drinks and medicines. Ask the children to find some. Make up a collection for the whole class. Get children to make a note of radio advertisements. Can they make a list of the different ways in which advertisers make smoking and drinking look attractive? What kind of people are in the advertisements? Why do tobacco companies often sponsor sports events? In what ways are some of the advertisements dishonest?

Can the children themselves design advertisements for newspapers or magazines or posters to illustrate for example:
- how much a smoker spends per year.

- the dangers of drinking alcohol and then driving
- the dirty aspects of smoking (smell, ash, teeth stains)
- the ill health which is caused by smoking
- the fires caused by smoking
- the poverty which can result when someone becomes an alcoholic

Can the children work out a small play, perhaps as a radio, film or television commercial. It could indicate the advantages of not smoking. It could stress the positive aspects (non-smokers are richer and fitter and they do not smell of stale tobacco).

Part II
Teaching and learning in health education:
the role of the school and the community

Chapter Eight

Methods, techniques, and lesson planning

A good teacher

To be a good teacher, you need to know:

- what you are teaching (the subject matter)
- how to teach it (the methods)

The chapters in Part I of this book contained some teaching suggestions. These suggestions showed how you could take knowledge about health and make it more interesting for children. In this chapter, we will concentrate on the methods of teaching about health. We will explain:

- the variety of methods which you can use
- how to plan lessons on health
- about links between health and other subjects
- how to check on children's progress

The most common teaching method

Think about the teachers whom you have known. Think about yourself teaching. What comes into your mind? You probably see a teacher talking at children. This is what most teachers do most of the time!

Perhaps for many teachers, the equation TEACHER TALKING = CHILDREN LEARNING applies.

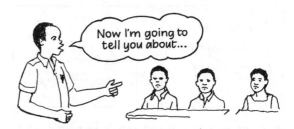

Now I'm going to tell you about...

Sometimes teachers have to talk. For example:

- You may want to give instructions
- You may want to explain an idea
- You may want to ask a question

But the problem is that the 'lecture method' is often the only method which teachers use. They stand at the front of the class with the textbook firmly in one hand while they TALK.

In this book, we have tried to suggest that there are other methods which you can use. Remember the old proverb:

> I hear and I forget,
> I see and I remember,
> I do and I understand.

Next time you teach, try to talk less! Get the children to talk more. Ask questions. Use some of the methods and ideas in this book. Remember that we receive most information about the world around us (about 70%) through the sense of sight. Use the children's sense of sight to help them to learn.

The most common visual aid

Most teachers have a blackboard in their class-rooms. Most teachers use the blackboard . . . but many do not use it well. Here are some simple rules:

- Write clearly, and in large letters, so that children can read what you write

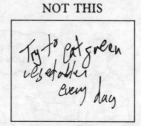

THIS	NOT THIS
Try to eat green vegetables every day	Try to eat green vegetables every day

- Write in a logical and tidy way so that children can understand what you have written

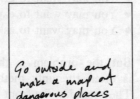

THIS	NOT THIS
1. Visit the compound 2. Note health hazards 3. Return to class 4. Draw a map of the compound 5. Show health hazards	Go outside and make a map of dangerous places

- If you have a big blackboard divide it as shown here, and do not scribble all over it.

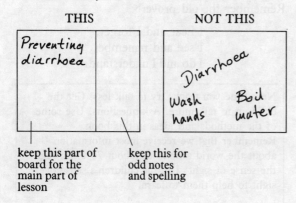

THIS

Preventing diarrhoea	

NOT THIS

Diarrhoea
Wash hands   Boil water

keep this part of board for the main part of lesson

keep this for odd notes and spelling

Organising the children

Many classrooms are like this:

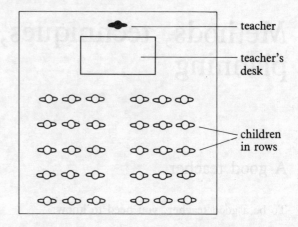

teacher

teacher's desk

children in rows

The teacher stands at the front. The children sit in rows in front of her. But that is only one way. There are many other ways in which to organise the children:

- The children (perhaps when they listen to a story) could sit in a semicircle around the teacher like this:

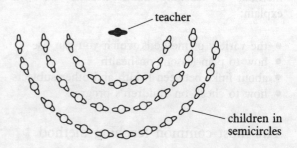

teacher

children in semicircles

- The children could sit in groups:

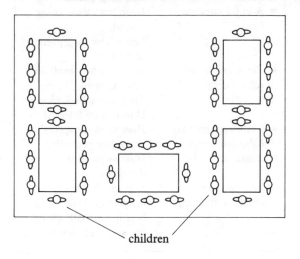

children

- The floor could be cleared for a drama and the children could sit around like this:

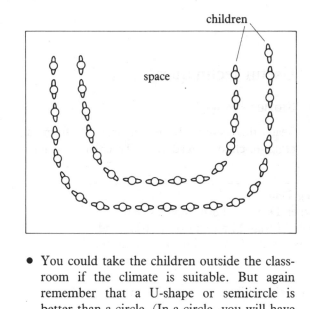

children

space

- You could take the children outside the classroom if the climate is suitable. But again remember that a U-shape or semicircle is better than a circle. (In a circle, you will have your back to some of the children.)

It is often a good idea to establish a routine with the children so that they will know what you expect them to do. Tell them clearly and quietly how you want them to sit. Good teachers rarely need to shout!

'Hidden' learning

This is not really a method of teaching but, especially in health education, it is important to know about it. Children do not learn from teachers only. They learn in many other ways: from their homes, from their neighbourhood, from the way that other adults (and other children) behave. This 'hidden learning' is especially important in the formation of attitudes. It is especially important, therefore, in health education.

What, for instance, do children learn from the situations illustrated here and over the page?

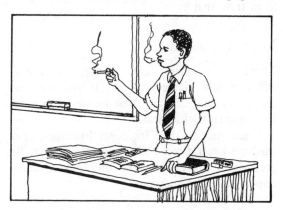

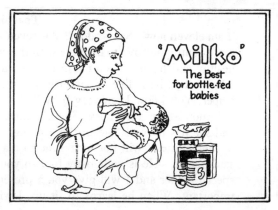

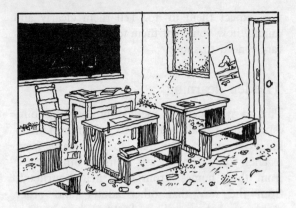

Large companies advertise their products. They hope to influence the choices which people make. Teachers, too, can advertise. They can advertise good health ideas by posters and displays. If the school environment is healthy then children will learn from that.

Incidental learning

There will be many times during school days when 'health' incidents occur. If you are alert and ready, you can use these incidents to teach the children useful ideas.

When you use real incidents like this, your teaching has a direct and immediate impact. Be prepared for occasions like these to reinforce important health messages.

Incident	Learning points
• A child cuts his finger	Keep cut clean, cover wound. Learn how to prevent in future
• Child arrives at school dirty	Dirty clothes smell and carry germs. They don't look nice. Skin can be infected.
• Child reports that baby sister has diarrhoea	How to make special drink (see page 91). How to prevent diarrhoea.
• Teacher sees children smoking	Explain about the dangers of smoking to health, and talk about the cost (see chapter 7).

Useful techniques

Stories

Read this story. It is an excerpt from a CHILD-to-child reader, 'Teaching Dani'.

Teaching Dani

'I am eleven now,' Sami said. 'I was seven when Dani was born. Mama said to me, "Sami, you have to help me with this baby! I want him to grow up strong and healthy and happy. I want him to learn to talk well. I want him to be ready for school when he is five. Your little sister can help, too, but you must be my special helper. You know I am very busy."

I know she is very busy. She is a nurse for sick children. She works in a hospital and she has to work late in the evening.

"Sometimes I will not have time to play with Baby, but that will not matter," said Mama. "He is your baby too, so you can play with him. You will be my special helper and I will give you a present each time Baby does something important. When he learns to sit up, I will give you some shorts. When he learns

---

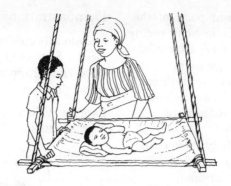

to walk, I will give you a shirt. When he begins to count, I will give you a special present." "But, Mama!" I said. "You don't need to give me presents. I want to play with Baby but I don't know how babies play."

"I will help you," said Mama. "I will tell you what to do. Do you remember how you learned to play football?"

"Yes, Mama."

"Do you remember all the things you had to learn? How to kick and how to pass the ball? Do you remember how you watched the other boys? You did what they did and you tried and tried."

"Yes."

"It is a little like that with Dani. He has to learn many things. He has to learn to use his body. He has to learn to use his arms and legs, his hands and feet. He must learn to make big movements, like sitting and walking. He must learn to make little clever movements like holding or catching or putting on his shoes. He must learn to use his eyes and ears, his taste and smell. He must learn to use his senses," said Mama.

"What a lot he has to learn!" I said.

"That is not all," said Mama. "He must learn to think. He must learn to use language. He must learn to talk and learn to listen. He must learn words and how to put words together. He must learn to ask questions."

"Can he learn all that?" I asked.

"Yes," said my mother. "He can learn it all if you help him and if we all help him."

"Yes, I will help," I said. "And you will help me. Will anyone else help me?"

"The other children can help you," said my mother. "They can play games with Baby. They can talk to him. Your sister can help you. The shopkeepers can help you. They can give you many things that they don't want. You can collect them for Baby to play with. The school can help. They can teach you how to make toys and games and books for Baby to play with. These toys and games will not cost any money."

That is how I began learning how to play with Dani.

What do you think is the main point of this story? How would you use it in your health lessons? Can you develop the story? How might Sami help Dani to walk or talk or count?

Children love stories. They can learn through stories. They are a powerful teaching technique. Learn to use them effectively! Remember:

- Work out the story carefully beforehand. Decide on the main message (or idea) which you want the children to understand.
- Write the story out or learn it before the lesson. Practise telling it before the lesson so that you can tell it well.
- At what point in the lesson will you tell the story? Decide this beforehand. Sometimes you can tell the story twice, perhaps at the beginning and end of the lesson. This will help the children to understand the point of the story.
- Prepare some questions on the story to check that the children have understood it. If the story is a long one, stop from time to time and ask questions. This will help to keep the children's attention.
- Children will enjoy a story more if you use pictures, or puppets, or a flannel graph (see page 154).
- Arrange the children so that they feel comfortable and can see you clearly.
- Tell the story in the children's own language. Keep the language simple.

Practise story telling

In many places in this book, we have suggested that you make up and tell stories. If you are in training, practise telling stories to each other. Choose an important health idea from this book and make up a story around it. Share stories with other students. Keep the ideas for when you are teaching in school.

Demonstrations

Occasionally children in Mrs Oyo's class get nose bleeds. She could **tell** the children what to do when this happens. But, instead, Mrs Oyo **shows** them what to do. She does a demonstration:

Cyprian volunteers to be a patient for the demonstration.

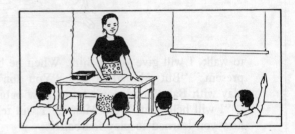

Cyprian comes to the front of the class. Mrs Oyo arranges Cyprian on a chair. She makes sure that all the children can see. Cyprian pretends to have a nosebleed. Mrs Oyo tells him to sit quiety.

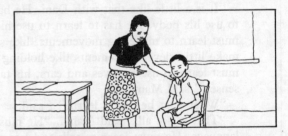

Mrs. Oyo shows the children how to pinch the nose to stop it bleeding.

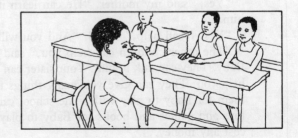

Now the other children practise on each other in pairs.

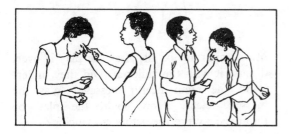

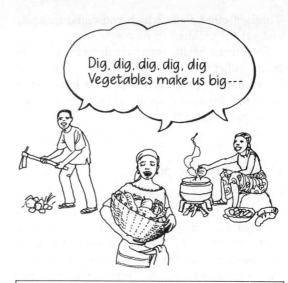

Think about this lesson

Mrs Oyo is a good teacher. She does not **tell** the children what to do for a nosebleed. She **shows** them. By doing a demonstration, the children can see for themselves what to do. Mrs Oyo takes care that all the children in the class can see the demonstration. She explains clearly as she does it. The children then practise the skill for themselves. This will help them to remember what they should do when someone has a nosebleed.

So remember
- Don't just tell! Show by means of a demonstration
- Make the demonstration clear
- Make sure that the children can see
- If possible, let the children follow the demonstration with practical action by themselves

---

Songs

Children enjoy singing songs. Songs can help children to remember an important health message.

Choose a well-known tune. Make up words to fit the tune. An example is shown here:

Let's eat three mixed meals a day,
Every day, every day,
Let's eat three mixed meals a day,
To keep our bodies healthy.

Let's eat wing beans every day,
Every day, every day,
Beans or meat stew every day,
To keep our bodies healthy.

Let's eat green leaves every day,
Every day, every day,
Let's eat green leaves every day,
To keep our bodies healthy.

Let's eat peanuts every day,
Every day, every day,
Peanuts, peanuts every day,
To keep our bodies healthy.

Let's eat fresh corn every day,
Every day, every day,
Corn with peanuts every day,
To keep our bodies healthy.

Let's eat fresh fruit every day,
Every day, every day,
Fruit will help us every day,
To keep our bodies healthy.

Think of other songs which you could make up and get the children to help you.

Sometimes health songs are broadcast on the radio either on programmes for health, or between other programmes. If your local station does not broadcast them, perhaps you could write and suggest the idea.

Drama and role-play

One of the most powerful teaching and learning techniques in health education is drama. When children act a play, they can identify with the characters in it. They learn the idea in a direct and personal way. In this book, we have often suggested drama or role play. (You will find examples on pages 122 and 135.

Here are some principles to remember:

- Make sure that the health message is clear.
- Prepare the plot of the play in advance. The children can help to work out the details.
- Decide how many children should have a part in the play. The others can either take part as the crowd or be in the audience.
- Make sure that everyone can see and that the actors have enough space in which to act.
- Discuss with the children what role each character should play.
- Decide with them how the play should end.
- Often children will need a few rehearsals of the play so that it runs smoothly. This is obviously necessary if the play will be performed to another class, to parents, or the community.
- The children will need to learn:
  to **speak in turn**
  to **face the audience** so far as possible
  to **speak loudly and clearly** (and only when the audience is quiet!)
  to **use costumes and props** (hats often identify a character or, if necessary, you could hang a label around the person's chest)

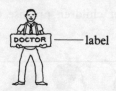
label

- Most important of all, after the play is over, discuss it with the children. Did they understand the main health message? Was the message clear? How could the play be improved? Were the actors convincing?
- Different groups could present the same play. For example, the teacher could divide the class into two or more groups. Each group then works out how to present the play. They then present the play in turn. There could be a discussion after each presentation.

(Children like puppets. They can perform plays using puppets. You will find ideas on how to make them on page 155.)

Present a play
Either with your fellow students or with children, prepare a play with a health message. Try to use the principles explained here. Ideas for plays may come from:

- the newspaper (a real life story)
- a problem discussed in a health lesson
- a picture or photograph illustrating a scene or problem

Discussions

In a discussion, the children should talk more than the teacher!
You may want to encourage discussion:

- after a story
- after a drama or role-play
- about moral issues (looking after disabled people, sex education etc.)

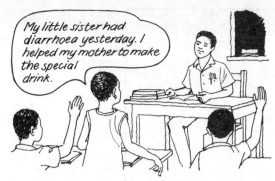

My little sister had diarrhoea yesterday. I helped my mother to make the special drink.

Children often expect the teacher to do all the talking. They may not know how to discuss. You may need to teach them. A discussion will be effective only if you have good discipline in your class. You cannot run a discussion if the children are noisy and do not behave well.

Here are some points to remember:

- Discussion is easier with older children.
- Children often try to talk at the same time. Teach them to talk one at a time. Teach them to listen to each other.
- Encourage quieter children to participate.
- Be a good chairman (chairperson). Steer the discussion. Make sure that children learn the health message. Make a summary at the end of the discussion of what people have said.
- Sometimes, you can divide the children into groups for a discussion. Appoint (or get the group to appoint) a chairman. The chairman of each group can then report back to the whole class later.
- You can start a discussion in several ways. You could use a picture or describe a situation. You could have a discussion after a drama or role-play. You could ask children about health incidents which have happened to them or to their families. Ask questions like:
What do you think should happen here?
What would you do in this situation?
What is the danger to health?
Do you think the people in the story acted in the best way?

Games

Like stories and plays, children enjoy games. Games can be useful in your health lessons. We have suggested games several times in this book. Games often introduce competition. Because of this, and because children like to win games, they concentrate on winning. Thus they may easily miss the important health message of the game. It is therefore very important to discuss the game with them afterwards.

Children have to learn to respect the rules of a game. This is an important thing for them to learn. It will help them to understand why a school has rules. Later, they will find it easier to understand about the laws (or rules) of their society and country. Sometimes rules prevent people from doing harm to themselves or others. This is why there are laws about road use or about taking drugs. Rules and laws should allow people to live happier and more healthy lives.

One good game which children like is 'Snakes and Ladders.' You can make up your own. You can make games with different health messages. One example is shown on page 152.

The rules are the same for all games of Snakes and Ladders:

- Two, three or four people can play.
- A player places a button (or seed) on square one. The buttons should be a different colour for each of the players.
- The players throw the dice. The one with the highest number begins.
- The first player throws the dice and moves his or her button forwards by the number of squares shown on the dice.
- If a player rolls a six, he can throw the dice again.
- If a button stops on the head of a snake, the snake swallows it. The player moves the button to the tail of the snake and reads the message there to the other players. That players's turn is now over. Next turn, he restarts from the bottom of the snake.

Snakes & Ladders

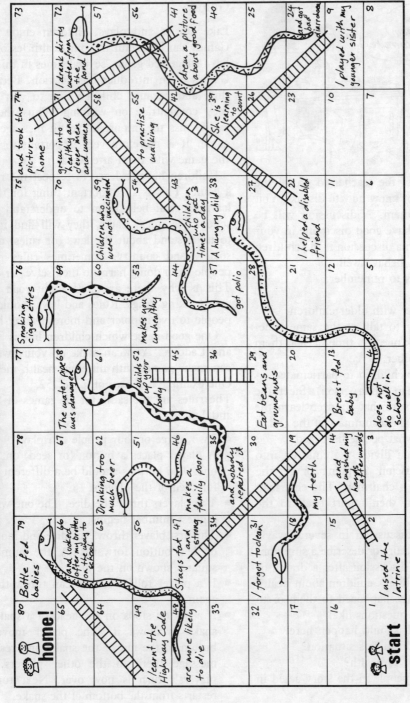

80 Bottle fed babies	79	78	77 Smoking cigarettes	76	75 and took the picture home	74	73
65	66 and cooked after my brother on the way to school	67 The water pipe was damaged	68	69	70 grew into healthy and clever men and women	71 I drank dirty water from the pond	72
64	63 Drinking too much beer	62	61	60 Children who were not vaccinated	59	58	57
49 I learnt the Highway Code	50	51	52 builds up your body	53	54 Children who eat 3 times a day	55 to practise walking	56
48 are more likely to die	47	46 makes a family poor	45	44 makes you unhealthy	43	42	41 drew a picture about good food
33	34	35 and nobody repaired it	36	37 got polio	38	39 She is learning to count	40
32	31 I forgot to clean	30	29 Eat beans and groundnuts	28	27	26	25
17	18	19	20	21 I kelped a disabled friend	22	23	24 and got bad diarrhoea
16	15	14 and washed my hands afterwards	13 Breast fed baby	12	11	10	9
start	2	3 does not do well in school	4	5	6	7	8 I played with my younger sister
				1 I used the latrine			

home!

- If the button lands on the foot of a ladder, the player moves it to the top of the ladder and reads the message to the other players. That player's turn is now over, and his next turn is from the top of the ladder.
- The first player to reach the last square wins the game. The player must throw the exact number needed to land on the last square (number 80 in the example shown).

Making and using teaching aids

Teaching aids need not be expensive. They can be collected and made by teachers and children. They can often be used again. It is useful if you have a cupboard or desk where you can lock them away. The following are some suggestions for teaching aids which may be useful during health lessons:

Pictures

Pictures give interest and colour to lessons. They can show the children something which they may not be able to see for themselves. You can use pictures when you are teaching the whole class, or you can use them for children's activities. These might be:

- games (where children match pictures with health messages)
- spot-the-mistake pictures (which show a deliberate health hazard)

You can get pictures for your health lessons from:

- newspapers
- magazines
- calendars
- advertisements

Or you could draw your own or get the children to draw them.

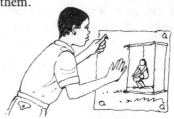

Try this idea!

In the West Indies, children at the top end of primary school drew some pictures. These illustrated an important health point. For example:

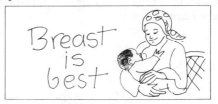

The children took the pictures home and showed them to their parents. They asked them to put them on the wall. In more than 75% of homes, the pictures were displayed. Parents who could not read particularly liked the pictures.

Remember, also, to put up children's pictures on the walls of the classroom. They like to see their work displayed. It makes the classroom more interesting. Pictures can remind children of important health messages. If possible, fix some wooden battens to the walls of the classroom. You can then pin the pictures to the battens. Encourage the children to look at the pictures. Change them as often as possible.

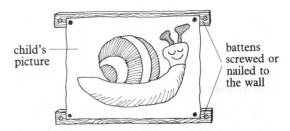

child's picture

battens screwed or nailed to the wall

Puppets

Children can make and use puppets in a play about health. Here are some ways to make puppets:

- they could draw a face on their fingers and nails

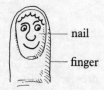

- or they could draw on paper wrapped around their fingers

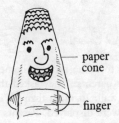

- or they can draw on matchboxes and put the matchbox on their fingers

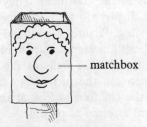

Handpuppets are more difficult to make but they last longer. The children can make the puppets and do the acting. They can speak the words just as in a play. You can see how to make them on page 155.

Flannel graph (or flannel board)

A flannel graph is a board which you cover with a piece of rough material. You can easily place pictures on it, and it is also easy to remove pictures. It is very useful in health education lessons (and in other lessons too). It can be made in the following way:

- get a board (perhaps made of plywood) about one metre square
- cover it with a rough piece of cloth or blanket
- stretch the cloth tight (pin it, or stick it behind the board)
- stick the picture (or words) onto card
- Stick flannel or sandpaper or soft cloth onto the back of the card. The card will now stick to the flannel graph. It can be taken off easily.

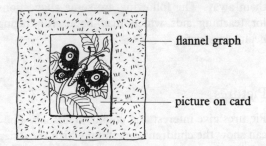

Use the flannel graph to illustrate stories and to give information. Remember to keep the pictures when you have made them. They will be useful again in the future. In what ways is a flannel graph more useful than a blackboard?

How to make a hand puppet (right)

154

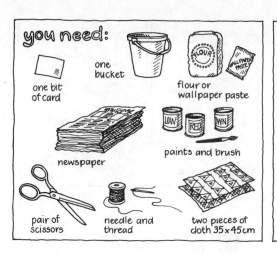

you need:

one bit of card

one bucket

flour or wallpaper paste

newspaper

paints and brush

pair of scissors

needle and thread

two pieces of cloth 35×45cm

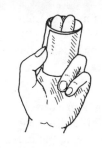

roll cardboard around your fingers and glue together to make the neck

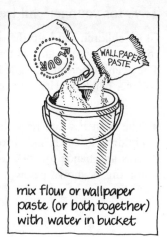

mix flour or wallpaper paste (or both together) with water in bucket

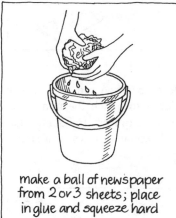

make a ball of newspaper from 2 or 3 sheets; place in glue and squeeze hard

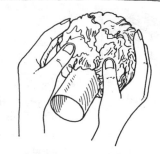

make hole in ball and put neck in; you can fasten neck to ball with paper and glue mixture

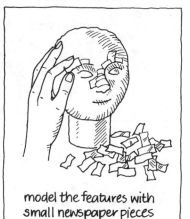

model the features with small newspaper pieces

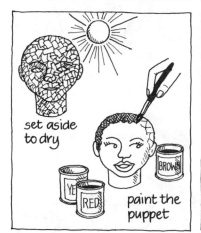

set aside to dry

paint the puppet

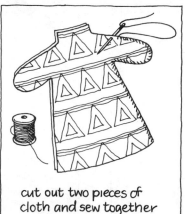

cut out two pieces of cloth and sew together

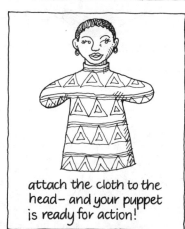

attach the cloth to the head— and your puppet is ready for action!

Toys for younger children

Older children can help the development of their younger brothers and sisters (see chapter 9). They can make some simple learning aids for the younger children. Here are two ideas:

- The bean bag can help three or four-year-old children to catch and throw. This helps their eyes and hands to work together. The picture for this is shown below.

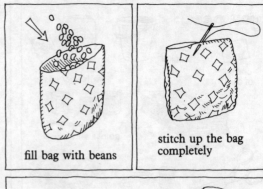

fill bag with beans

stitch up the bag completely

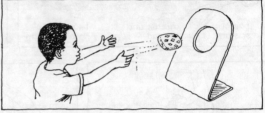

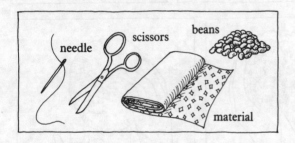

needle scissors beans

material

- Dominoes made of bamboo can help five or six-year-old children to match the number of dots. This helps them to learn to count. They also learn about keeping to rules in a simple game.

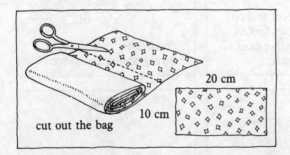

cut out the bag

20 cm

10 cm

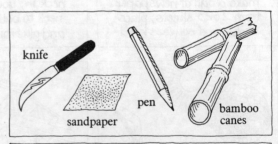

knife

sandpaper

pen

bamboo canes

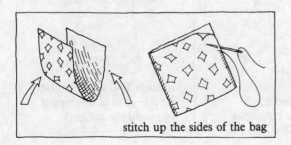

stitch up the sides of the bag

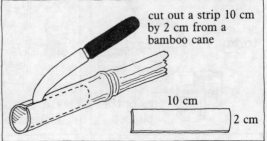

cut out a strip 10 cm by 2 cm from a bamboo cane

10 cm

2 cm

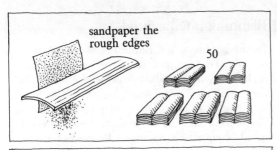
sandpaper the rough edges

50

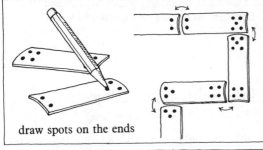
draw spots on the ends

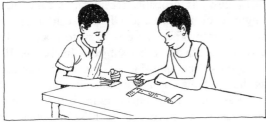

Planning health lessons

Planning is important. In health lessons, as in other subjects, you cannot teach good lessons unless you prepare well. Some lessons need more preparation than others. Even a few minutes thought and preparation will improve how you teach.

Here are some questions to ask yourself when preparing a lesson:

● Is there a curriculum or scheme of work?

If so, what work has been covered? What do the children already know? From what point should the lesson begin?

● What do you hope that the children will learn?

What are the objectives of the lesson? Think about what you will teach and what the children will learn. Try to be as specific as you can. For example, consider these objectives for a lesson on malaria:

Objective: To teach children about malaria.

Objective: Children will learn what malaria is, how it is caused, and how we can prevent it.

What do you think of these two statements? Which is a better statement of an objective and why?

● What subject matter will you cover?

This should obviously be related to the objectives of the lesson. Don't be too ambitious! Remember that children need time to learn new ideas. Choose subject matter which is relevant to their age, understanding and experience. Think about the major health problems where you live.

● What materials and equipment do you need?

Make any visual aids which you will need. If the children will do any activities, think about and collect the necessary materials. If possible, keep a stock of junk materials in your classroom (boxes, tins, paper, bottles, jars, wood).

● What methods will you use?

Think about the subject matter of the lesson. Think about the variety of methods which you might use. For example, a lesson on keeping clean might include the following:
- discussion about need for a clean body
- a story about a child who was always dirty
- questions about the story
- demonstration on how to wash, cut nails, and comb hair
- children practising these activities themselves

157

- questions about the lesson
- at home: how to help younger brothers and sisters to keep clean

Think how you will organise the children (in groups, as a class, or for individual work).

It is often useful to make a short lesson summary for yourself. This will remind you about the lesson sequence which you have planned. You can take the summary into the classroom.

● **How will you end the lesson?**

It is not always easy, but try to leave time so that you can end the lesson well. There are three points to consider.

First, how much have the children understood? Ask them questions about the lesson. Prepare the questions which you will ask. (See the section 'Checking up' later in this chapter.)

Secondly, do you want the children to do some activity or preparation before the next health lesson? For example, you may ask them to:

- identify health hazards at home

- play with their younger brothers and sisters

- discuss a health matter with their parents

- write a few sentences about a health topic

- make or bring something to school (such as a comb, a finger puppet, crayons to colour a picture)

Make it clear what you want them to do. Don't forget in the next lesson to check that they have done it!

Thirdly, tell the children what they will learn in the next lesson. That means that you need to know what the lesson will cover. (See chapter 10 on how to plan a scheme of work for health.)

Links with other subjects

Health is only one subject in the primary curriculum. It probably receives less time than language or mathematics. Health can often be brought into other subjects. Try to make links between health and other subjects. In chapter 10, we discuss the question of 'class' or 'subject' teachers. How you make links between subjects depends upon the system operating in your school. How can you improve these links if you are a 'subject' teacher for health? You might like to discuss the problems involved.

In **mathematics**, children learn to measure and count. For example, they may measure their growth in height, or count their pulse and breathing rates. They may weigh themselves (and other children) if scales are available. They may do traffic surveys. They may keep records of accidents. They can learn to display this information in tables, bar charts and graphs.

Science and health science are closely linked (sometimes health is actually included in the science curriculum). Modern science teaching in primary schools often emphasises the skills or processes of science (observing, classifying, . . . and so on). These skills can be useful also in health science. For they are thinking skills. They are skills which are useful throughout life.

There is much subject matter which is common to both science and health science. Consider, for example, knowledge about:

- the body and how it works
- diseases
- food and nutrition
- effects of smoking on the body
- the importance of sanitation

Make sure that there is coordination on the teaching of these topics.

Language skills are important for most of the other subjects in the curriculum. Children need to be able to speak, listen, read, and write with confidence. Remember that when you are teaching health you are also teaching language. Similarly, in language lessons, you can select subject matter about health. Let children write stories about health topics. Let them listen to stories and create role-plays. Bring health ideas into language lessons.

Physical education (PE) and health are often formally linked in the primary school curriculum. You can use the opportunities which PE lessons present for teaching about several important topics. For instance, you could talk about:

- first aid
- importance of exercise and keeping fit
- learning 'motor' skills
- fairness in sport and competition (keeping to the rules)

Other subjects such as art and craft, creative activities and moral education all present opportunities for links with health education. Discuss these links with other students or teachers.

Checking up

You teach so that children will learn! It is clearly important to know whether children have learnt something and what children have learnt. In fact, you need to check on their progress, to evaluate their learning. Particularly in health education, you also want to know if children apply what they learn. For example:

- Do they come to school cleaner?
- Do they clean their teeth more regularly?
- Do they use the latrine at home? Do they use it properly?
- Do they apply what they have learnt about treatment for diarrhoea?
- Do they discuss health problems with their parents?
- When they look after younger brothers and sisters, do they apply their health knowledge?

Checking up in the lesson

Here are some methods which you can use:

Question and answer technique

You can get some idea of children's understanding by asking questions to the whole class. Let all the children think about the question.

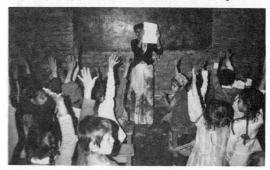

Ask them to put up their hands if they know the answer. Now point to an individual child and see if he can tell you the answer. This encourages all the children to think about the question. It is a better way of checking up than if all the class shout the answer together. However, by this method, it will take a long time to check the learning of all the children in the class.

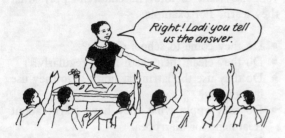

Right! Ladi you tell us the answer.

Assessing individual children

Sometimes you will want to know how individual children in the class are progressing. Which children in the class do not understand the work? Which children find it too easy? Do any need special help?

Perhaps the most obvious method is to give the children a written test. But remember that this is of no use unless it is corrected! The children need to know how they have performed. If your class is large, correcting a written test may take a long time. Sometimes you must mark children's papers yourself. But there are some ways to save your time. You could ask children to exchange papers. They then correct each other's. The children thus receive immediate feedback on how they have performed. They should **learn** during this process.

However, you do not have to give a written test to assess children's learning. Watch individual children during health lessons . . . and at other times. There are probably some who particularly excel in:

- role-play
- looking after younger brothers and sisters

- drawing pictures
- discussions
- being kind to disabled children

Keep a note of this information for future references.

A quiz

To make a change from the usual written test, you can set a simple quiz. For example:

- put foods (or pictures of foods) around the classroom
- number each one
- now ask the children to name each one and write whether it is GO, GROW, GLOW or STAPLE

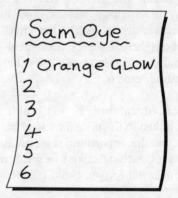

Sam Oye
1 Orange GLOW
2
3
4
5
6

Perhaps you could offer a small prize for the child who gets the most correct.

Beyond the classroom

It is quite easy to check whether children can remember a simple fact. It is much more difficult to check that they have understood and apply this knowledge. Particularly in health education, this application of knowledge is important. Health education is effective if, as a result, the children, their families, the school and the community are healthier.

For example, you teach about **accidents**: therefore accidents to children on the road or at home should decrease.

You teach about **diarrhoea** and how to prevent it: therefore fewer children should get diarrhoea.

Here are some ways to check if children are applying their knowledge:

- Older children could keep **health diaries**. In them, they record good health practices which they have followed. For example, they could record about:
keeping clean
looking after others
preventing disease
preventing accidents
eating well

   Check their diaries from time to time. Ask children to read aloud from their diaries to the rest of the class. Is there evidence that they are applying their knowledge?

- **Looking and listening.** Ask younger children about their health practices at home. Watch them at school. Look and listen for evidence that they apply what they learn.
- **Health scouts.** Older children could be health scouts (see page 198). They could report on health hazards in and around the school. This could be an after-school activity as in some schools in Kenya and Sudan.
- **Parents and community.** Read chapter 11 of this book. Encourage parents and others to come to the school. Talk to them about health problems. Is there any evidence that the children take home ideas which they have learnt in their health lessons?

Assessing your own lessons

Try to assess your own teaching performance! Particularly if children have not learnt well, think about your teaching. How could you improve? You may need to:

- try different activities
- use different or additional materials
- organise your class in a different way

The following checklist may help you:

- Were the children interested in the health topic? Was it close to their experience?
- For how long did I talk in the lesson?
- Did I ask the children questions? Did I listen to their replies?
- Did I use any aids? Could the children see them? Were they interested in them?
- What did the children *do* in the lesson?
- Was there a variety of activity?
- Did I try to check what the children had learnt?

Try to be critical of your own teaching performance. Your health lessons will improve . . . and your pupils and the community will be healthier.

Chapter Nine

CHILD-to-child

Here is a story:

A special friend

Akin is four years old. He has a brother, Sam, who is two years old. His mother is expecting a baby soon. Akin and Sam are often left alone when their mother has to do some gardening. But they are never afraid because they have a friend. This friend is a very special person.

When Akin had diarrhoea, his friend gave him a drink made from salt and sugar. When Sam cried, she comforted him and played games with him. She often plays games with Akin and Sam. Sometimes she tells them stories. When their mother is away, she gives them food and teaches them how to clean their teeth. She shows them how to wash their hands before eating. She shows them how to wash the cooking pots afterwards. When Akin is older, he wants to be like his friend.

Who is this friend? Is she a teacher or a health worker or a doctor?

One day, she showed the two boys a place where it was dangerous to play. There were pits in the ground, and long grass everywhere. She told the boys that there may be snakes there. She told the boys that nasty insects called mosquitoes lived there. If they bit the boys, the mosquitoes would give them an unpleasant sickness called malaria. She said that the teacher at her school was asking the local council to clean up this place and cut the grass.

The boys' friend wanted to know if they had had an injection when they were babies. She asked their mother about this. Akin wondered for a long why she wanted to know this. One day, his friend explained that her teacher wanted to know about who had had injections.

Why? Who is Akin's and Sam's friend? Who is this person who cheers them up, plays with them, helps them when their mother is busy and tells the school teacher about them?

It is Martha, the girl who lives in a nearby house. She goes to the local primary school. She has learnt how much she can do for children who are too young to go to school.

What is CHILD-to-child?

This chapter is about children like Martha. It is about how older children can help and care for younger children. We call helping and caring activities like these, CHILD-to-child activities.
We write the first word in capitals to show that we are talking about an **older** child caring for a **younger**.

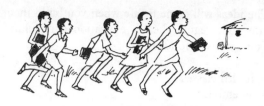

children going home

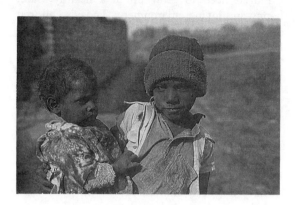

The children who you teach in school, or will teach, could be like Martha. They could learn from you useful knowledge and skills about good health. They can pass these on to their younger brothers, sisters and friends who are not at school. As a teacher, you are probably in a better position than anyone else to introduce children to the CHILD-to-child idea. In fact, many of the suggestions in this book can be used by older children in caring for younger.

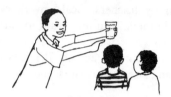

older children helping younger

CHILD-to-child began as a programme for the International Year of the Child in 1979. Since then, the programme has produced:

- a book
- many activity sheets
- a series of readers
- a manual for the handicapped
- a manual for those who run refugee camps
- other materials

You will have already noticed that we have referred to CHILD-to-child ideas many times in this book. We used this symbol to draw your attention to them:

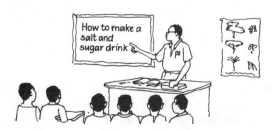

teacher teaching in school

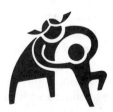

The ideas will come to life when you build them into your regular health education curriculum. You can use the ideas in:

- health classes
- assemblies
- out-of-school education
- cooperation with the health worker or doctor

In some places, CHILD-to-child programmes are run by teachers, health workers, scout leaders and others. You may want to participate in these or you may want to fit CHILD-to-child into your own teaching schedule. It is a flexible idea! Take it and use it as it suits you.

Why CHILD-to-child?

In many parts of the world, older children (like Martha in the story above) care for younger children. Often families are large. Mothers have to cope with the new baby. In this situation, older children in the family have to accept responsibility for the younger children. CHILD-to-child is a reality. It exists already. Teachers and others can build on this reality. You can use CHILD-to-child to reach children:

- who have not yet gone to school
- who may never go to school

Thus, older children can provide the channel through which we can reach the world beyond the school. It is a world where the health needs of young children are great.

As you will know from reading this book, we now have the knowledge to help children to be healthy. It is life-saving knowledge. Throughout the world, young children suffer from:

- diarrhoea
- malnutrition

- malaria
- measles
- polio
- bilharzia
- hookworm
- disability
- injuries caused by accidents
- many other diseases and health problems

Children need to grow up in a healthy, safe, happy and loving environment. Today's children are tomorrow's parents. Today they may be looking after their younger brothers and sisters. They are learning what it means to be a parent. In particular, they can:

- learn to recognise signs of common illnesses
- learn when to send for help and when they themselves can help
- learn what to do for diarrhoea
- tell the teacher if their brothers and sisters have not been immunised
- help to prepare balanced meals
- teach younger children how to keep their bodies, hands and teeth clean
- teach younger children road safety
- help to prevent accidents at home
- play games with younger children and make simple toys for them
- help children who are disabled

Thus, older children can help to meet the health needs of younger children. However, as teachers, we should recognise that CHILD-to-child has a wider message for us. For it is a most powerful idea. It is an idea which reaches beyond health education. It can change schools, our role as teachers and our view of the education process:

- CHILD-to-child encourages cooperation and caring. So much of life in school is about competition and exams.
- CHILD-to-child is practical and about the real world. All children in school know younger

children and most will have younger brother and sisters. Many already accept the responsibility of looking after them. CHILD-to-child is directly relevant to their lives.

- CHILD-to-child is about children learning from each other and teaching each other. It is about sharing knowledge and skills.
- CHILD-to-child helps the school to reach towards the community. It brings school, parents and community closer together.
- CHILD-to-child encourages children to realise that they can play an important role in helping with the health of the family. They will learn that they are valued not merely as future adults. They are people in their own right who can make a real contribution to the health of others and themselves.

Reaching children who do not go to school

In many places, there are older children who do not go to school. Maybe they have to help their families at home. Perhaps they have to help the family to earn a living. They may have to look after their younger brothers and sisters. Sometimes the children who do go to school can pass on good health ideas to these older out-of-school children. This is quite a long chain! Remember that messages can be distorted as they pass from one person to another. Thus, it is important that the teacher makes the original message clear and simple.

> **Make health messages clear and simple!**
> Stand or sit in a circle. One person makes up a message and whispers it to the next person. He or she then whispers it to the next and so on around the circle. How does the original message change? It is important that the original message should be clear and simple.

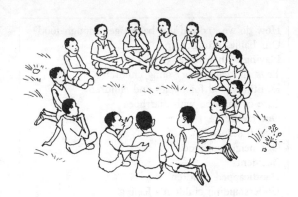

How does CHILD-to-child work?

Many of the ideas in this book can be passed from older to younger children. When you are teaching about health, ask yourself:

- Can the idea be used by older children in caring for younger?
- Is it knowledge which is useful for younger children?

If so, then draw the attention of the class to it. Remind them about CHILD-to-child. Ask them in a later lesson whether they shared the idea with their younger brothers and sisters. Did they play with younger children? Did they help those who were sick? Did they look out for ways of preventing accidents?

The activity sheets produced by the CHILD-to-child programme best explain how it works. The full list of titles is shown on the next page.

How do we know if our babies get enough food?
Our babies growing up
Playing with younger children
Toys and games for young children
Healthier food for babies and children
Care of children with diarrhoea
Our teeth
Health scouts
Our neighbourhood
Accidents
Handicapped children
Understanding children's feelings
Looking after eyes
Let's find out how well children can see and hear
Caring for children who are sick
Early signs of illness
A place to play
Helping the severely deaf child
Growing vegetables in containers
The management of little children's stools

Examples of CHILD-to-child sheets

We give on the following pages examples of these activity sheets:

1 'Caring for children who are sick' describes how an older child can comfort and care for a younger child who is sick.
2 'Playing with younger children' explains that, for healthy mental development, children need to play. Older children can learn how to play with babies and young children.

Finally . . .

Remember that these activity sheets are examples of how the CHILD-to-child idea may be used. We give other examples elsewhere in this book. Look particularly at:

Other activity sheets are available from the programme. CHILD-to-child materials are available through TALC (Teaching Aids at Low Cost), Institute of Child Health, 30, Guilford St, London WC1N 1EH, England.

A word of warning!

Remember that some of the ideas which children bring home from school may not agree with the beliefs and practices of parents. This is a difficult problem. As a teacher, you can help children to cope with this situation by working together with parents. At open days and parents' meetings you can explain what the school is trying to do. Teachers, head teachers and health workers need to work with parents and in the community.

Caring for children who are sick

This sheet can be used with
'Early Signs of Illness'

The Idea

When a young child is sick, the family may be worried. An older child can help to comfort and care for the sick child until it gets better. The children also help the mother if she is working or very tired.

What can the older child do for the sick child:

Liquids: the sick child needs to *drink a lot*. The older child can give him *clean drinks* such as weak tea, juices or soups. If he is passing a lot of stools and vomiting, he may need the special drink for diarrhoea.

Food: although the sick child may not seem to be hungry, he should be helped to try to eat. *It is very important* that sick children are given some food to help their bodies fight the illness. A sick child who has no food becomes weaker and will take longer to get better. The older child can help to prepare soft mashed foods such as banana, paw-paw or beans with a little oil added. It is often better to give *many small meals*. Help feed the sick child but be careful that he *does not choke*.

Comfort and care: the sick child needs to rest in a *quiet, clean* place. Where possible, let light and fresh air in, but *keep away* flies, insects and animals. If it is very hot, fan the child or bathe with a cool, damp cloth. If the child is *vomiting* help him to lie *on his side*. Then he will not choke on his vomit which can be dangerous. Children who are very sick and *do not move much*, need to be turned regularly. The older child can rub the *elbows, heels* and *buttocks* from time to time to prevent them for getting sore. If the child is having *great* difficulty in *breathing* he may feel more comfortable if he is raised up rather than lying flat.

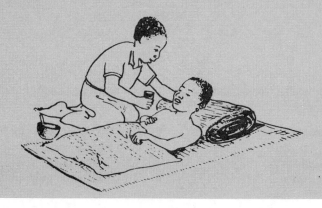

It is very important to comfort the sick child with words, stories and songs. It may even help if the older child holds him. He needs to have someone with him. If the sick child has a *very high fever* it might help to *bathe* the body with a soft cool and damp cloth. *Do not wrap* the child's body tightly with many cloths or clothes. This makes him hotter and may increase the possibility of fits and brain damage from very high temperature.

Remember: when the child starts to get *better* he needs *extra* foods, liquids and care. He will go on needing help until he is quite well again.
But keep babies and small children away from sick children if possible.

Cleanliness

Another thing the older child can learn is how to keep the sick child clean.

Clothes: when a child is sick, he sometimes vomits or passes water and stools where he is lying. The older child can help by taking the dirty cloths and clothes and washing them in a separate place as soon as possible. Keep them away from the rest of the family washing and places where people draw water for drinking.

Skin: it is important to wash the sick child's skin with clean, warm water. This stops it from becoming dirty and infected and making the child more ill. If the child wants to scratch the skin, try to help it not to damage itself.

Eyes, *nose* and *mouth*: these should be kept as clean as possible by bathing with *clean, cool water*. This will prevent more infection. If the mouth is sticky or dirty from vomit it can be rinsed. A little cooking oil can be used to moisten dry and cracked lips.

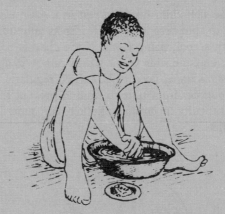

Activities

The teacher or health worker can ask the children questions about how if feels to be sick. For example:

- When were you ill?
- How did you feel?
- What did others do for you?
- When did you feel better?

- Has any other child in your family been ill?
- Who looked after him?
- What did your mother say?

Children should be shown the correct way to sponge and wash a sick child. They can be encouraged to practise on a doll or on each other.

Ask children to press their elbows on the table, desk or door for a few minutes then see if the elbows feel sore. This will help to explain pressure sores.

One child can have its temperature felt by placing hands on the forehead. The child can then be wrapped up in clothes tightly for a time. Ask the child how he now feels and see if his forehead feels hotter.

Food can be mashed and passed down a tube of bamboo or through a narrow necked bottle. Let the children see how soft food goes down easily whereas hard or lumpy food sticks.

Find out who cares for sick people locally and how they do so.

A play or story can be acted to show how others cared for a sick child. Or one child can show other children what he did when one of the younger children was ill at home. Or several children play the part of all the people in the family and show what they do when a little child is ill.

Card games, posters and strip cartoons can be made by the children to show the stages of an illness and what care was given.

How did the activity work?

- How many children have looked after a sick child and what did they do?

- Children can keep diaries or medical cards to record how they helped.

- One child can be asked to pretend to be sick. Other children can act or mime how they can care for him and comfort him: for example, wash his clothes, help him eat, give him many drinks, bathe his head and hands – rub his elbows and so on.

- Quizzes can be used a few months later to see how much the children have remembered.

Who can use this activity sheet?

- Teachers in school can use the ideas in health lessons for short dramas and mime.

- Health Extension workers can use the ideas with groups of children in the village, in a queue, at the health clinic, in youth groups or in schools.

- Youth leaders, Scouts and Guides may wish to adapt these activities and award badges or a certificate.

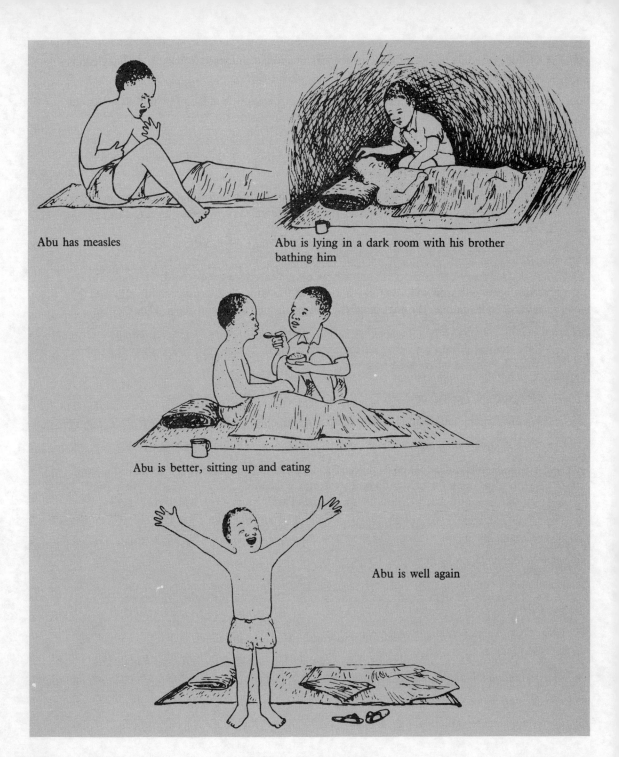

Abu has measles

Abu is lying in a dark room with his brother bathing him

Abu is better, sitting up and eating

Abu is well again

Playing with younger children

This sheet needs to be read together with the sheet 'Toys and games for young children'. This sheet talks about *why* children need play to develop and *what kind* of play children can provide for each other. The second sheet concentrates on *materials*: where to get them, how to make them, how to use them.

The idea

Children everywhere spend some time looking after their younger brothers and sisters, and this is one of the most important ways in which they help in a family. Children will often be told what *not* do do when looking after baby – '*Don't let her near the fire. Don't let her hurt herself.*' But they are seldom told what to do. Yet if a baby is not played with she may grow up not being able to learn properly. This activity is to help older children learn how to play with younger children so that babies will grow up bright and alert.

Who introduces the activity?

Whoever introduces these ideas to older children needs to explain *why* children need play as well as *how* play can be organised. They need to explain the ideas to parents and help gain community support, particularly when older children help with play groups and child-minding groups. Many different people and means can be used to introduce the activity: schools and school teachers, health workers at clinics and in homes, youth leaders, and even the press and radio.

Children and play

Older children can observe young babies in their household. Discuss with them the 'play' of young babies. What can they do at different ages? What makes them laugh? What makes them move their hands, their heads, their legs?

How can we help them learn to do more things? Here are some ways. Children may suggest others.

Young babies

These need to be handled as much as possible. They learn mainly through being touched. Young babies like to look at things. They will look at a hand moving slowly in front of them, or a mobile hung above their bed. They enjoy people hiding their face suddenly behind a corner or a piece of cloth. Young babies like to listen. They like to hear the sound made by stones rattling in a tin can. They themselves can play with a dry seed pod or other things that make a noise when rattled. They will turn to discover where hands are being clapped. But *most important* they like to be talked to. We should always talk with baby and encourage her to talk back. The sounds she makes are her own language, and language is perhaps the most important thing for baby to learn.

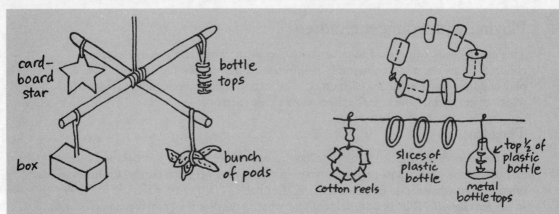

A hanging mobile for a baby to watch

Things for a baby to play with

Babies learning to crawl

As well as other activities, babies like to learn to use their bodies. Put them on their stomachs so that they can push themselves up. Help baby to sit. Put things just out of reach so that he has to find them. Give babies spoons, sticks and noisy things like pans and tins to hit. Give them things to pick up and play with. Always talk with them and encourage them to imitate words. Put into words what you are doing. They will start to copy you.

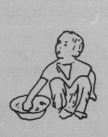

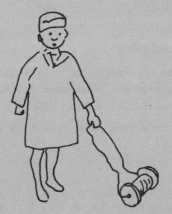

Babies learning to walk

Help baby to stand. Be ready to catch him when he tries to walk. Babies like to be thrown carefully up and down. Take them for small walks, show them things and talk with them about what you see. Give them things to push and pull. Toddlers like to do things. Have them help when they are being dressed. They can learn to talk about their clothes and what they are doing. Give them matchboxes or tins with seeds and stones they can remove. They like to climb into cardboard cartons and hide behind chairs.

Young children not yet ready for school

At this age the child is very active and always learning. She needs to be given a lot of challenge through many different kinds of play and an older child can do this. Older children may talk about young children they know. They can try to remember about themselves when they were younger. What can young children do for themselves at different ages? What things do they like to do on their own? With other children? What games do they play? What new games can we teach them?

Different kinds of play

There are many different kinds of play. The older children can talk about games from their own area and discuss: *Who plays them? – boys? girls? babies? Are they played alone? – in pairs? in groups? Do they need materials? – a special place?*

Water, sand or mud

Given a few materials children can play with water and sand for hours. Provide different sized tins, gourds and calabashes. Put holes in some of them. Paw-paw, banana stems and bamboo make good pipes and gutters. Tins, seed pods and pieces of wood make boats. Hollow reeds and soap can be used to blow bubbles.

Building games

Maize cobs, match boxes, scraps of wood can be used by children for building. Soft pith from palm fronds, grass stalks and thorns are used for constructing. Sisal bark and other materials can be used for weaving.

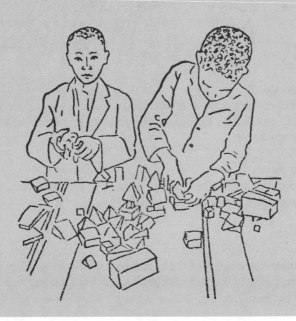

Sense games

Scraps of cloth, shells, almost anything can be put into bags for children to identify by feel only. Scraps of soap, onion, flowers and so on can be wrapped in pierced pieces of paper to identify by smell only. Objects can be put into tins to identify by sound only, when the tin is shaken.

Pretend games

Children love to play mother or father or teacher. Try to provide a variety of materials that children can use to make these games more interesting – for example, materials for making house, preparing food, making dolls, playing at shopping.

Activity games

Children like to run and play tag games. Fallen trees and steep banks are good places to climb and to slide down. Simple swings can be made. Old tyres are good to roll and to climb through. Stilts can be made with big tins and string. Large stones can be placed so that children have difficulty stepping from one to the other.

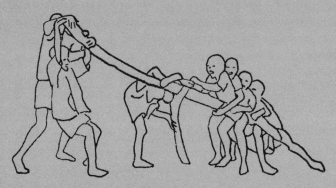

Learn what adults do

Small children will enjoy a visit to a workshop, bakery, etc. to see work being done by the adults in their community. Encourage the children to talk about what they have seen when they come home.

Taking things to pieces

Children learn from finding out how things work. Old pieces of cars, broken clocks, locally made animal traps, anything safe will do.

Playing with the sun

Children can play tag with their shadows. They can draw round their shadows in the dust. They can make the shadow of their finger point at stones. They can make their shadows stand on, carry, kick other children's shadows. Children can play games with mirrors or shiny pieces of tin.

Other games

Many other games are played that children can learn from. Flying kites, playing with tops and hoops, clapping and counting-out games, hop scotch, skipping and other similar games are good for children to play.

Riddles, songs and stories

Language development is very important. The stories, songs and riddles which children learn give them confidence in using language. They also help the children understand their culture and its values.

Organising play

Older children will need to think of the ways in which they can help younger children at home, at school and around them to play better. There are many places in which they help:

- at *home*, where children already play, older children can be encouraged to make a special place. They can have a special box for baby's play materials;

- *in creches*, *nursery groups*, older children can be encouraged to help the nursery school teacher by making materials for play;

- *at school* older children can be encouraged to organise play areas and materials for the younger classes;

- at *clinics* and other meeting places the older children can help by providing play materials for young children attending with their parents.

If the children want to help organise better play for younger children they will need to know how to go about it by:

- talking things over and planning how to bring play materials into their homes;

- discussing with the nursery school teacher and the childminder how best to help;

- persuading the Headteachers and community members that the school or meeting place can be used to set up a play activity.

Chapter Ten

Organising Health Education in school

This chapter is about how to organise health education in the primary school. We shall consider:

- the responsibilities and problems which a primary school teacher may face
- organising the staff resources in school
- planning the scheme of work
- how to help the school and its children to be healthy
- how to cope with sick children

Tackling the right problems

Some schools are big. Some schools are small. Some are in big cities. Some are in country villages. Some schools are near a hospital or good dispensary. Some schools are far from the nearest doctor or health worker. Every school is different. The health problems are different in different places. Thus you will need to adapt the suggestions in this book according to your situation and circumstances. If the school is near a busy main road, you may need to pay particular attention to road safety. If many babies in the area die of diarrhoea, you may need to teach children about the sugar and salt solution (see page 91).

The problems faced by primary school teachers are often great. It is important to distinguish problems which, as a teacher, you can help to solve. If you tackle problems which are beyond your reach, you may become depressed and even bitter. If, however, you tackle those problems which you can solve, you will develop in confidence. You will be ready to face fresh tasks. Your success will enable you to move forwards. You will realise that you can help to make better lives for the children in your care. You will be able to help your fellow teachers to understand what they can do for the health of the children.

So remember!

make small changes
and you will cross
the river successfully

run too fast . . .
and you will
fall in the river

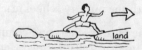 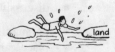

On being a primary school teacher

It is not easy to be a good teacher. There are many pressures to face. First, there is the problem of **isolation**. Teachers are often isolated professionally in their classrooms. They are between the four walls of the room with forty, fifty or even more children. They do not often see how other teachers teach. They may not often be visited by other people such as the head-teacher, parents or other teachers. The school may be a long way from the next nearest school. The inspector rarely comes. When he does come, he may be more interested in routine administrative matters than in what happens in the classrooms. The opportunities for in-service training may be rare. There may be few books or other resources in the school. In such circumstances, where do you as a teacher look for help? How can you learn to do the job better? Who can advise you when you have a particular problem?

Primary school teachers are often expected to be able to teach the majority of subjects on the curriculum. This can be a difficult task for many teachers. You may enjoy teaching language and social studies, for example, but be much less confident about science, mathematics and health education. Teachers have a big responsibility. The children will learn through you: through **your** knowledge, skills, and attitudes.

Organising the staff resources in school

Within the school, it is the head-teacher who can have most effect in easing some of these pressures and solving some of the problems. He can encourage policies and ideas which will help teachers to help each other. For example, he can encourage teachers to:

- visit each other's classrooms
- watch each other teach
- take joint classes (team teaching)
- form a club, perhaps with other teachers from nearby schools
- pass on ideas learned during in-service training to other teachers
- share the work of curriculum planning for the school

Perhaps most important of all is the policy on specialisation. Who is in charge of health education for the school? In many schools, nobody is in charge! Each teacher may be expected to teach the subject as part of the regular curriculum. It may be that the teachers do not talk to each other or to the head-teacher about health education. Of course, a teacher who is in charge of the subject does not have to teach this subject to every class. But it does mean that she takes a special interest in it. She has certain jobs and responsibilities. For example she can:

- Help other teachers in the school. She can give them advice and suggest teaching materials.
- Attend in-service training courses on health education and pass on what she learns to her colleagues at school.
- Develop with the head-teacher a scheme of work in health education for the school (see page 178).
- Keep the head-teacher informed about health matters in the school.
- Be responsible for the health of children in the school.
- Be a member of the local community health committee (see page 196).
- Develop links with the local health worker or hospital.
- Teach some health education lessons in other classes in the school.

Thus, this teacher becomes the most important person in the school for encouraging the development of health education. But she cannot do all the work herself. Many of the other teachers will also have to teach the subject. It is her job to help them to teach it better, to be a 'resource' person, and to build their confidence. The head-teacher can play a most important part here. He can provide the essential support to the health teacher. He can enable her to work cooperatively and effectively with her colleagues.

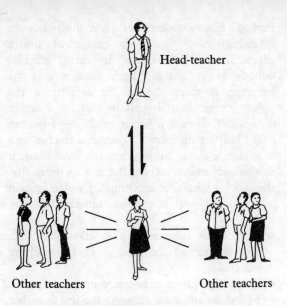

Head-teacher

Other teachers

Other teachers

Health teacher

On health matters, the health teacher also has the main contact with any supervisors or inspectors, and with the local education authority.

Schools and countries differ in their policy on specialisation. Limited specialisation, as described above, has worked in many places. It is useful not only in health education but in other subjects too. However, it is particularly important in health education where it is so important to share knowledge with the community.

Planning a scheme of work

It is important to have a scheme of work for the school. The scheme will be the 'blueprint' for the head-teacher, you and the other teachers. A blueprint is a plan. It gives you a framework. It means that you and other teachers have some idea of the **scope** and **sequence** of the subject matter which will be covered. (Scope means the range of content. Sequence means the order of

teaching that content.) Without a scheme, it is difficult to have proper coordination between teachers. The result may be that children are taught the same thing over and over again as they pass through the school. Or they may omit to learn some important knowledge or skill.

There are two situations which you may meet:
1 where there is a national, regional or state syllabus 'curriculum,' or 'scheme of work'
2 where there is no official syllabus or scheme

1) Where there is an official syllabus or scheme

Many countries of the world have centralised education systems. Policies and curricula are decided by 'the centre' (by national or regional or state government). The schools are expected to put them into practice. In health education, this may mean that a national syllabus has to be followed. Sometimes these syllabuses are very detailed. They may indicate exactly what subject matter should be covered during a particular year or term. They may even suggest certain methods that should be followed. Sometimes the syllabuses just indicate the content to be covered. Others translate the syllabuses into behavioural objectives. That is to say, they state how the children's behaviour should be changed as a result of studying the topic.

Let us examine two health syllabuses, one from Papua New Guinea, one from Nigeria.

A health syllabus from Papua New Guinea
On page 179 is an overview of the syllabus from Grade 1 to Grade 6. There are six themes:

- Health and disease
- Personal health (clean body)
- Family health (clean home)
- Community health (clean village)
- Mental health (a happy life)
- Social well-being (a useful life)

Papua New Guinea health syllabus

Health Overview

Theme	Grade 1	Grade 2	Grade 3	Grade 4	Grade 5	Grade 6	Theme
Health and disease	World health / World diseases	Living things / Friends and enemies	The body, the mind / Living together	Living things and man	A concept of disease	Disease and its effects on human growth and development	**Health and disease**
Clean body	What is clean? / What is dirty?	How is the body kept clean and strong?	Physical well-being	How the body works	Personal hygiene and health	Decision-making and personal health	**Personal health**
Clean home	A clean home / A dirty home	What helps to make a clean home?	A good, safe, clean home to live in	The family – food and nutrition	Family hygiene and health	Family health, living in a changing society	**Family health**
Clean village	A clean village / A dirty village	What helps to make a clean village?	A good, safe, clean village to live in	Living together	Community hygiene and health	Community living and community health protection	**Community health**
A happy life	Working, playing and health	Man has a mind	A happy life	Living with change	Mental health / The mind, body and behaviour	Decision-making and responsibilities for mental health	**Mental health**
A useful life	Helping ourselves and others	More ways to help ourselves and others	A useful life – our place in the home and village	Living in groups	Social problems, responsibilities and health	Citizenship	**Social well-being**

For each grade, the content which the teacher should cover is summarised. Here is the summary for Grade 5:

Summary

1 Health and disease	food and health – weight charts, underweight children, the right foods, balanced meals, malnutrition, food for babies, older babies, food for mothers, breast feeding, dangers of bottle feeding, meals for school children, food problems in your area.	**4** Community hygiene	your community towards a healthy community diseases of young people old people
2 Personal hygiene	cause of disease physical fitness games clothes cleanliness healthy teeth personal appearance every day is health day	**5** Mental health	how we change how we learn mental growth praise and blame behaviour the healthy person the place of the person in his society
3 Family hygiene	our family village houses and town houses fresh air and sunshine beauty in the house useful things in the house the cooking area a safe house	**6** Social well-being	courtesy and manners tolerance community teamwork social problems ignorance and disease education for life

A health syllabus from Nigeria

The syllabus for health education in Nigerian primary schools lists the content which teachers should cover on a class-by-class basis.

A syllabus for Primary Three is shown on the next page.

Nigerian primary health education syllabus

First term: **Primary Three**

1 Personal health

   (i) personal cleanliness and grooming
  (ii) care of the eyes, ears, nose and teeth
 (iii) need to alternate work and play
  (iv) choice and care of clothing

2 Communicable diseases

   (i) common diseases of the school-age child in Nigeria
  (ii) dangers of diseases to health
 (iii) how disease spreads
  (iv) how to prevent the spread of diseases

3 Community health

   (i) sources of community water supply – good and bad sources
  (ii) how to keep the community clean
        (a) regular collection and removal of refuse
        (b) clean toilet habits in the community
 (iii) individual responsibilities for community health
  (iv) advantages of clean homes in clean community
   (v) the available health services in the locality

4 Current health problems (as the need arises)

Second term:

1 Nutrition education

   (i) kinds and sources of food in our locality
  (ii) the basic food groups in Nigeria: energy-producing, body-building and body-repairing food
 (iii) care of foods
  (iv) good eating habits (such as table manners)

2 Safety education

   (i) common accidents
  (ii) where, when, and why accidents occur
 (iii) how to avoid accidents
        (a) at home
        (b) as pedestrians
        (c) at school
        (d) at parties

3 Current health problems (as the need arises)

Third term:

1 Mental and social health

    (i) why we should know our limitations
    (ii) how we choose our friends
    (iii) how to get along with others at home, school, and at any other place
    (iv) what we have to do when we have problems
    (v) our duties to our neighbours, classmates and friends

2 Family life and sex education

    (i) my home and my family (differences in Nigerian context)
    (ii) family living in the locality (a description of family set-up)
    (iii) children's duties in the home
    (iv) boy-girl relationships (at home, school and community)

3 Body structure and functions
    (i) the human body as a bicycle or motor car (reference to parts and harmonious workings)
    (ii) why all parts of the body should be taken care of
    (iii) how to maintain a healthy body
    (iv) my responsibility for a perfect working of my body organs

4 Current health problems (as the need arises)

In some ways, an official syllabus may be helpful. The content is laid out for you and you work your way through it. You know where you stand. There is a sequence which you and other teachers can follow. However, there are also disadvantages. It is difficult for a national syllabus to be suitable for every part of the country. It may be designed for town schools but not those in rural areas. It may be too wide-ranging in content. It may require you to teach things which you do not consider important.

A syllabus does not necessarily have to be taught in the order in which it is laid out. Syllabuses, which have been wisely prepared, encourage local modification and adaptation. So, even if there is an official syllabus, **planning by the school is essential**. A syllabus has to be shaped into a scheme of work with which teachers feel comfortable. It has to be adapted to the circumstances of your school. If there is a health education teacher, the main responsibility for this lies with her. She will consult with the head-teacher and the other teachers. In some schools, the head-teacher will assume this responsibility.

Try this exercise:
1 Look again at the syllabus from Papua New Guinea. Choose a grade/class level other than Grade 5 (say Grade 2 or 6). Make a summary table similar to the one for Grade 5. Show in the table what content you might include under each of the six themes.

2 How would you alter the syllabus from Papua New Guinea to suit the particular circumstances in your country and local situation?

3 Look again at the syllabus from Nigeria. What main themes are covered? Suggest how these themes might be developed in later grades, say 4 and 5.

4 How would you improve these syllabuses?

2) Where there is no official syllabus or scheme

If there is no official syllabus, then responsibility for planning the scheme of work rests entirely with the school. Again, the head-teacher or health education teacher will take the lead, but always in consultation with other teachers. Here are some questions which might be asked before a scheme of work is developed:

- What **resources** are available? Is there a sympathetic doctor or health worker near who is willing to visit the school and to provide advice? What other sources of knowledge, information, and skills are available – books, people with first aid qualifications, a knowledgeable supervisor or secondary school teacher, for instance?

- What is the **context** of the school? Is it urban or rural? How big is it? Does the head-teacher attach importance to health education?

- What are the most serious **health problems** in the area? How can the school help to resolve them? Is there an awareness in the community of health problems?

- What is the **time allocation** for the subject? Is it taught as a separate subject? Or is it taught with physical education? Is this laid down nationally or can the school decide? Is there a daily or weekly **health review** of the children, perhaps on a class basis?

With answers to questions like these, it is easier to develop a more relevant and teachable scheme. Probably the best way is to proceed step-by-step:

- Decide on the subject matter. Use the ideas in Part I of this book. Remember that little children can remember and understand only a certain amount of factual information.

- Children's understanding of an idea develops slowly. You cannot teach them about accidents in Grade 2 and think that you have covered that topic for ever. Children should meet the idea again later when they are older and more responsible. The school can develop and extend their understanding in later years. Gradually, they will build up their understanding and knowledge. However, this is not easy. 'Spiralling' like this can become a boring process of repetition. Children may feel that they are not learning anything new. As you develop a scheme of work you will need to build in progression. Both in content and methods, you can indicate how the same general subject should he treated differently as children get older. For example:

Topic	Grade 2	Grade 4	Grade 6
Accident **Content:**	Accidents that have happened to me	Dangers at home and school	Coping with accidents
Methods:	Discussion	CHILD-to-child	Simple first aid in
	Drawings	Looking around school	practice
	Story	Writing about hazards	A play about accidents
	Road safety	at home and school	
		Road safety	

- Make an outline of the scheme. Discuss it with the head-teacher and other teachers. Make sure that they agree with its scope and sequence.
- Then develop it further. Try to produce supporting material which indicates not only what to teach but also how to teach. Other teachers can help. They can tell you how activities went and where they found problems. What was successful? Have they got any ideas which can be shared with other colleagues?
- The scheme need not be fixed and final. As every teacher gains in experience, new ideas can be incorporated. However, it is probably sensible not to change the general structure drastically every year! Your colleagues need time to learn new ideas. So, when there is a scheme which teachers like and understand, keep it.

Make the school a healthy place

It is important that the school is a healthy place. The health teacher has the main responsibility for this. But the head-teacher, other teachers, and the local inspector can all help him or her to put these ideas into practice.

Water

A good water supply is important for good health. It is best if the school has a piped water supply. But in many places, this may not always be possible. If piped water is not available, try to have a clean well in the school compound. Keep a bucket of water or a tap near to the latrine to encourage children to wash their hands. A pot of clean drinking water can be kept in each classroom.

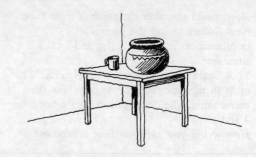

Washing hands

Children should learn to wash their hands:

- after using the toilet
- before they eat

They should understand that this is to prevent the spread of germs which cause diarrhoea and typhoid. However, they cannot learn this practice unless water is easily available. If there is no pipe water, you can use a bucket with a tap at the bottom like this.

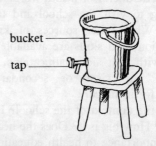

You may have to teach young children how to wash their hands. If possible, they should use soap. First, they should wet their hands, then rub in soap, then rinse with water. Rinsing with water is better than nothing.

Sanitation

It is important that the school is a clean place. It should be a **model**. It should be a place where children learn clean habits. It will only be a clean place if teachers insist on high standards of sanitation. Remember the facts about the spread of disease (see chapter 5). Disease can be spread by flies and other insects, water, and the faeces of animals and people.

Look at the school illustrated here. Decide how the sanitation in a school like this could be improved.

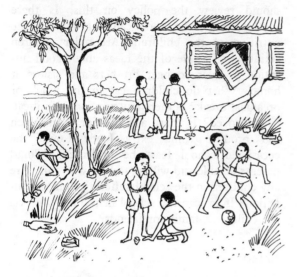

Try to encourage the following practices:

A school toilet
- Make sure that there is a suitable toilet and that children know how to use it. A toilet which can be flushed with water is obviously best, but is often not possible in many rural primary schools. It may be necessary to build a pit latrine.

Here are instructions for building a pit latrine:

1 Find a piece of ground at least twenty five metres from the school building and the source of drinking water. If possible, choose a place below the water source. Otherwise the latrine may pollute the water and make people ill.

2 Mark out a circle on the ground about one metre in diameter.

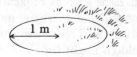

3 Dig out the pit, about two metres deep.

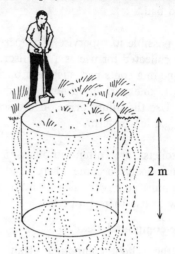

4 If possible, make a woven mat (from bamboo for example) about one metre in diameter and two metres deep. Put this inside the hole. It will help to prevent the sides of the pit from collapsing.

5 Make a cover for the pit from strong planks or bamboo. The hole in the middle should be about forty cm long and about twenty cm wide.

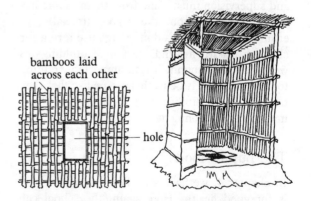

bamboos laid across each other

hole

6 Make a hut to fit over the latrine. The appearance will, of course, vary according to the materials locally available.

7 Keep the pit latrine clean. Put earth or dry

leaves on from time to time. Then it will not smell so bad.

- If it is possible to supervise it properly, urine can be collected for use as a fertiliser. Collect the urine in a container, such as a bucket, and dilute it: one part of urine to four parts of water. Use the dilute urine on the soil in the school garden or farm.

School toilets are often unpleasant places! They can easily become dirty and smelly. Teachers must supervise them. Children should learn how to use them properly.

Keep the compound clear

- Keep the school compound clean. Have a special place for rubbish. Bury in a pit rubbish which cannot be burnt or made into compost.
- Cut the grass and keep it short. Use the grass, old leaves, and manure for the compost heap.

Get the children to help

It is not necessary for the teachers to do all the work to make the school a clean and healthy place. But the motivation, example, management and supervision must come from them. Time has to be allocated from the school timetable to ensure that cleaning is done. Organise a rota for cleaning classrooms and the school buildings as well as the compound. It is an important training for the children. It helps them to realise that they have a responsibility for the state of their immediate environment.

The pupils' food

In chapter 4, we have seen how important food is for good health. Here again, the school can encourage children to put these ideas into practice. The pattern will be different everywhere according to the school's situation and practices. For example, many schools may make no provision for lunch or breakfast. Some may encourage local traders to come to the school to sell simple food to the children during breaks. Some may suggest to parents what food the children should bring. Some may even be able to provide food. From time to time, the school staff should review the policy on this. Is there anything which the school can do to improve the nutrition of the children? Are older children taking home some of the ideas about good nutrition to their younger brothers and sisters at home? What do children eat in the lunch or breakfast break? Is there any way in which it can be improved? Is there a garden or farm which can produce some extra food? Could the occasional school feast be organised? Would parents be able and willing to help with this? Are any children in the school suffering from malnutrition? If so, can the school help directly or via the children's family or friends?

Safety

Look around the school for possible safety hazards. Pay particular attention to the following:

- Road safety: is the school near a main road? Have the children been warned about the dangers of fast-moving traffic? Have they been taught practical road safety (see chapter 6 for some ideas)? Is there a fence? Do the children know about the dangers of playing on or near a main road? Is there anyone who can help young children to cross the road before and after school?
- Dangerous play equipment: check that seesaws, swings, and ropes are kept in good order.
- Health scouts: use the health scout idea (see chapter 11) to check around the school for possible hazards such as broken glass and tin cans, stagnant water where mosquitos and other insects can breed, dirty toilets, places where children might slip.

- Cooking facilities: if cooking is done, check that the arrangements are safe and clean. Particular care is needed if water is boiled in large pans.

Help children to be healthy

The suggestions above are about general health matters in the school. But, as a teacher, you also have to consider the health of individual children.

A health review
- Consider having a morning health review each day or perhaps twice or three times a week. This might be during the school assembly or in individual classes. All teachers will need to help with this. An actual inspection may not be necessary but it is important to watch for any sick children. If there is a creative activities period, this may be a good time to observe children. Watch, too, for children who have not come to school. They may not have come because they are sick. If the children live near you, you could visit the parents to find out what is wrong. Or you could ask other children who live near to visit the family.

Check how well children can see
Watch for children who may not be able to see well. Look out for the child who wants to sit near the front of the class in order to see the board. Look out for the children who squint.

Here is a quick way to make an eye chart to test how well children can see. The method described is useful for children who may not be able to read well. If children can read well, then make the chart using many different letters.
The chart is shown on this page.

1 Make the E's according to the diagram. Make them the right size. A stencil may help. Cut

out the E's and glue them onto the chart. Older children could help.

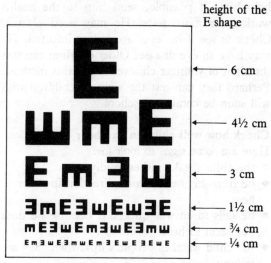

height of the E shape

6 cm

4½ cm

3 cm

1½ cm

¾ cm

¼ cm

the size of the E gets smaller and smaller

2 Make another large E shape out of cardboard or other stiff material.

3 Hang the chart where the light is good. Make a line about six metres from the chart. The child being tested stands behind this line with the cardboard E.

4 Either the teacher or another child points to the shape on the chart. The one being tested must hold up his E in the same direction as the E being pointed to:

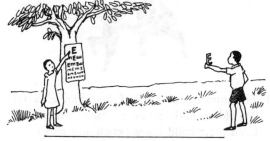

6 m or 20 feet

If the child can read the bottom three lines easily, then he sees well. If the child has difficulty reading the top three lines, then he sees poorly.

If he sees poorly, make sure that he sits near the front of the class. Encourage his friends to help him. If possible, send him to the health worker for more tests. He may need glasses. Check to see if his eyes are red or infected. He may have an eye disease. Older children can test the sight of younger children using this method. Perhaps they can test the sight of children who will soon be coming to school.

Check how well children can hear

Here are some signs to look for:

- the child speaks rather loudly
- he turns his head in one direction in order to hear
- he fails to answer questions because he does not seem to hear
- the child watches people's lips when they are talking
- sometimes a child appears to be quiet, sullen, even rude (it may be that he does not hear well and needs help)

As for testing sight, it may be a good idea to test children's hearing, particularly when they first come to school. Here is a possible way to do it, using older children as helpers:

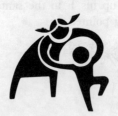

1 The children being tested stand in a semicircle. An older child stands by each younger one. Each older child has a pencil and paper.
2 An older child stands at the centre of the semicircle. He should be several metres from the younger ones.
3 The older child then calls out the name of an animal very loudly.

4 Each younger child whispers the name to his helper who writes it down.
5 The older child again says the name of other animals. Each time he says the name he makes his voice softer, until he is whispering.
6 The young children tell their helper what they hear. The helpers write it down.
7 After about ten animals, the helpers compare their lists to see what the younger children have heard.

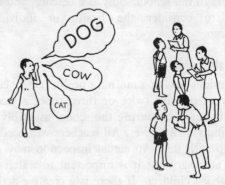

If any child has heard fewer names than others, he may have a hearing problem. Let him sit at the front of the class. If possible, he should be examined by a health worker especially if he has pus in an ear or frequent earache.

Check that children have been immunised

- Make sure that children have been immunised. The serious diseases against which children can be protected by immunisation are described on page 87. The local health worker or doctor should be able to cooperate with the school to ensure that an immunisation programme is organised at the school. Care will be needed to manage such a programme as the polio vaccine, for example, has to be given three times. Careful records should be kept.

Remember mental health

- The mental health of children is important. Watch out for children who are very slow at their work. They may need special help. Encourage other children to help them. Even though it may be difficult for you, try to make time to give them individual attention, (see the suggestions in chapter 3).

Even for normal children, school can be a frightening place, especially when they first come to it. The head-teacher and the other teachers are the people who can do most to create a happy, caring atmosphere. Remember that children copy what adults do, not what they say! They use adults as their models. The circumstances around a child determine what he learns and how he behaves.

> A child who lives with CRITICISM learns to CONDEMN
> A child who lives with HOSTILITY learns to FIGHT
> A child who lives with RIDICULE learns to FEEL SHY
> A child who lives with SHAME learns to FEEL GUILTY
> A child who lives with TOLERANCE learns to BE PATIENT
> A child who lives with ENCOURAGEMENT learns to HAVE CONFIDENCE
> A child who lives with PRAISE learns to APPRECIATE
> A child who lives with FAIRNESS learns JUSTICE
> A child who lives in SECURITY learns to have FAITH
> A child who lives with ACCEPTANCE AND FRIENDSHIP learns to FIND LOVE IN THE WORLD

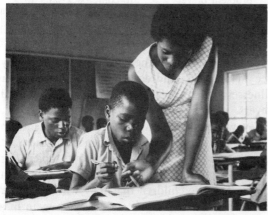

Good teachers pay attention to individual children

So, as a teacher, you can help to create this caring atmosphere. You can encourage the children to be kind and tolerant towards each other. There may be many opportunities to do this during the day:

- in activities lessons, children can learn to work in groups
- in physical education classes, children can learn fairness in sport
- at break times, children can learn to play together. (Remember that it may be necessary to supervise these break times. If children quarrel, they may need the help of adult teachers.)

Helping sick children

Sick children may come to you for help. Or you may notice that a child is ill. What will you do? Whether you like it or not, you may be the person who must decide what to do about a sick child. This situation is the more likely if your school is remote. If a school is a long way from the nearest doctor or hospital, you may often be the person who must decide what to do.

This book cannot tell you how to be a doctor. It cannot tell you about the variety of illnesses which may effect children. Nor is it a book about first aid. However, it can help you to make decisions about how sick a child is. Break the problem into two parts:

(1) First, ask: **What is wrong with this child?** In fact, you have to make a **diagnosis**.
(2) When you have made a diagnosis, you can ask yourself: **What shall I do about it?**

If you approach the problem in this systematic way, you will feel more confident. Gradually you will gain experience. You will be able to recognise children who are seriously ill. You may be able to save a life. You may help to reassure children who are frightened.

189

What is wrong with this child?

You can gather information to help you to answer this question in two ways: by **questioning** and by **observation**.

Questions are essential. They help you to focus attention on what might be wrong. Let us consider an example. A child comes to you complaining that he has a pain. Ask him these questions:

- Where do you have the pain?
- How long have you had the pain?
- Have you had the pain continuously?
- Have you had the same pain in the past?
- Does the pain come at any special time? (For example, does it come in the night, after eating food, when you run?)
- How bad is the pain?
- Is the pain getting worse or better at the moment?
- Have you had any other complaints such as cough, headache, fever?

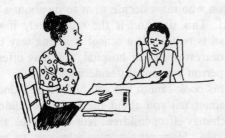

With answers to questions like these, you will begin to understand if the problem is serious or not. Is the child describing a pain which is serious? Does it demand immediate attention? Or is the pain perhaps psychological? Is he worried about school work or life at home?

While you ask these questions, observe the child. Ask yourself:

- Does he look ill?
- Is he feverish? (To see if his temperature is high, feel the forehead.)

- Is he in pain?
- Is he short of breath?
- Is he anaemic? (A pale pink tongue and a pale inside of the lower eyelid are symptoms of anaemia.)
- Is he dehydrated? (Symptoms of dehydration are sunken eyes and skin wrinkled like an old person.)

What shall I do about it?

By now you will have some information. You will have some answers to your questions and you will have observed the child closely. If you feel that it helps, write some brief notes. With this information, you can decide what to do with the child. Here are some of the possibilities which may be open to you:

Condition	Action
1 Seriously ill	Send to hospital immediately
2 Could be seriously ill	Send to health clinic, doctor, or hospital, as soon as possible
3 Ill, but not seriously	Will probably get better by himself, possibly some simple treatment necessary
4 Not ill, emotional problem or very minor sickness	Reassure child, ask him to come back later if not better

Number 3 is perhaps the most difficult. You may see many sick children. Most will have minor illnesses. These include coughs and colds, mild fevers, mild attacks of vomiting and diarrhoea. They will get better without any treatment. In fact, there is no treatment for most of them. It is most important not to give out tablets for them. If you do, children will come to expect them. Tell the children that they will get better soon. Tell them to come and see you again in a week if they are not better.

If you send a sick child to hospital or to the health worker or to a doctor, always send a letter with him. Explain what you think the problem is. Mention if you have given any tablets (such as choloroquine for malaria). If you think that the problem may be emotional, say this in the letter.

A final word of warning

Always remember that you are not a doctor! You are – or will be – a teacher. When children come to school, they are in your care. You should think of yourself as an intelligent parent who can recognise a genuinely sick child. You are the person who can 'filter out' (identify) these children and decide what to do with them. Think of yourself in this role. Don't pretend to be a doctor!

Never give or suggest medicines whose effects and side effects you do not know or understand.

Chapter Eleven

School and Community

Your personal example

A good teacher is a person who points the way to others. You can point the way towards a healthy life by the type of life which you lead. This is particularly important if you live in a small village or community where everybody knows you. As a teacher, you will be a rather special person in that village. Both children and adults may think of you as a **model** – as somebody to copy. Thus, it is very important that your way of life is worth copying.

First, take care about your personal appearance. If you are clean, healthy looking, and tidily dressed, people will listen to what you say about health matters. They will copy you and try to be like you.

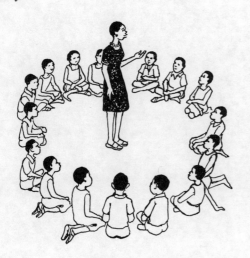

Secondly, there is your own home. If your home is clean and healthy and you follow the other practices suggested in this book, people will copy you. They will see that not only do you talk about being healthy, but that you **are** healthy.

Thirdly, in school time take special care to set a good example. In particular, don't smoke!

Begin with your own family!

As a teacher, you are to some extent a public person. You will be observed and judged by the children and adults where you live. Because of this, your family needs to understand your responsibilities. Help your wife (or your husband), your relatives, and your children to have the same attitude towards healthy living as you yourself have. Thus, a good place to begin in health education is with your own family. Help them to understand your job as a teacher, and why you recommend certain practices. You have read about many of these practices in this book. If, for example, you live in a place where malaria is common, then you should give your children anti-malarial tablets until they are five years old.

A note to women teachers with children

Do you have a baby? If so, continue breast feeding until the baby is two years old. We have seen that this is a very important way to give children a good, healthy start in life. **The best food is breast milk.** Weaning foods can be introduced at six months, but breast feeding should not be stopped. Breast milk and weaning foods can be given together. It is important that births are spaced properly. If children are born close together, their health may suffer. Their mother's health suffers. The whole family suffers. Perhaps you live in an area where sexual intercourse is not expected for several months after the birth of a child. After that time, you may wish to use contraceptives if they are available. **Try to leave a birth interval of between two and three years.** Your whole family will be healthier, and a good example to the rest of the community.

You probably want to return to work soon after you have had a baby. Naturally, you may want to continue to earn money. Perhaps you ask your mother or another relative to come and look after your baby. If you are in this situation, give your baby breast milk in the morning and at night. Remember that breast feeding:

- is good for the emotional security of a baby
- helps to protects a baby from infection

The best person to look after a baby is its own mother. The child benefits from close contact with its mother, and will have a better start in life. Obviously, if you are working, you will give special attention to birth spacing.

People help to sell their goods by advertising. You can help to sell good health by advertising. You can advertise your healthy family! In a tactful way, tell your colleagues in school about the practices which you follow. Talk to other people in your community about their families. By using your own family as an example, you can influence the way that people think.

Sometimes it is important to remember that other people may not be able to follow your example. As a teacher, you may be a richer member of the community than other people. For example, it may be that you follow the good practice of sleeping under a mosquito net. But other people may not be able to afford mosquito nets. In a situation like this, it is most important to be tactful. For instance, it may be wise not to teach children that they must sleep under mosquito nets in order to keep healthy. Their parents may not be able to afford mosquito nets, and a conflict will be created between them and their parents.

To summarise these principles:

- Be clean and tidily dressed both in the classroom and at home.
- Keep your home clean and tidy.
- Follow the practices which you teach your children.
- Encourage your family to be good examples to the other children and adults in the community. Remember, especially, that older children can be models for the younger.
- Don't expect or encourage people to adopt practices which they cannot afford.

The teacher and the community

Teachers are often expected to be leading members of the community in which they live and work. This can be a big extra burden in addition to the work which has to be done in school. However, it can also be satisfying to know that your special skills and knowledge can help people towards better, healthier lives. It is often much easier to be a part of a local community in small villages or towns than in big cities.

Teachers probably do not think of themselves as **experts**. But when they have been living in a place for some time, they do become experts in many ways. They have special knowledge and experience of the local community and environment. They can have a good influence on the health of the whole community. Doctors are usually found only in the big towns. There are not many doctors. They often live a long way away from country villages, and small towns. They may not know the local area well. But teachers **do** know the local area. They can help people to enjoy better health.

Let us assume that you have been teaching in a particular area for some time. What special knowledge and experience do you have? First, you understand people's beliefs and customs. You probably speak the same language. You may even have been brought up in the same village or at least in that area. You have sympathy with people's problems.

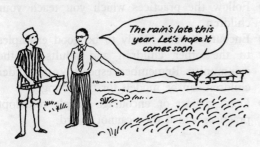

The rain's late this year. Let's hope it comes soon.

Secondly, you know the children in the community, and their parents. You may come to know those who have particularly health problems (disabled people for example). For some children in particular, you may know the family background well.

Thirdly, you know what people eat. You know what foods are available at certain times of year. You probably know how people could have diets which are better balanced, given the food which is grown and is available.

Finally, you know the common health problems. You know which are the most important diseases and what people die from. You may also know some useful medical 'folklore'.

With this special knowledge of your area, and your skills and experience as a teacher, it is possible to contribute to a healthier community. Certain principles are important. A community can become healthier:

- when people in it **understand** better what their problems are and how they are caused
- when they **communicate** with one another and discuss what they can do to make their lives better
- when they **act** to improve community health

Some suggestions for action

Let us see how it is possible for teachers to help in translating these principles into practice. Remember always, that it is essential to get the support and enthusiasm of the head-teacher for carrying out ideas like those listed below.

Bring the parents, and other adults, to school

Too often, the school is seen as a place for children and teachers only.

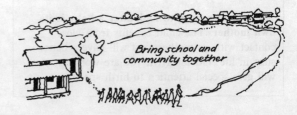

Bring school and community together

Involve parents in the life of the school. Otherwise, there is the danger that children learn one thing at school and something quite different at home. For example, at school children may learn to wash their hands before eating. Then they go home, and they see their mothers preparing food with dirty hands. Who should they believe? Their teacher? Or their mothers? This sort of experience makes them confused. The school points them in one direction, their homes in another. Of course, it is not possible to reach all the adults in the community. But many can be influenced through informal visits of parents (at the end of the school day for example). Or you could hold special open days when parents are invited to the school. This is chiefly a question of **attitude**. If the school looks **outwards** to the community, parents will come to it. If the school looks **inwards**, parents will not come. They will be frightened and stay away.

There are many ways in which the adults in the community can be used in a health education programme. Encourage these people to take part in school life wherever possible. Here are some examples.

The Medical Assistant or Community Health Worker

(These people have different titles in different places). Ask him to come to the school and explain his job to the children. Ask him to tell them about the diseases which he treats, and how he treats them. What are his main difficulties? How was he trained? When should the children come to him?. These are some of the questions he could answer. Perhaps the children could pay a visit to the dispensary and see him at work.

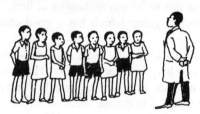

A Doctor or Nurse from a local hospital

If your school is in a town, a doctor or nurse could make a visit. Perhaps they could give a talk or demonstration on First Aid. Or they could discuss the running of a large hospital.

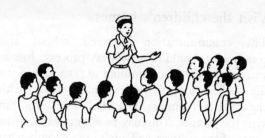

The Village Chief or Leader

If any community effort in health education has been (or will be) organised, such a person can be very helpful. They can encourage children to take part in the programme, and explain how it will benefit everybody. They will understand better the problems of teachers and perhaps become more interested in the school's role in the community.

The Community Development Officer

It is important to encourage his interest in the school. Perhaps he can arrange for community effort to improve the appearance of the school compound and sanitation. He can explain to the children about health projects in which they can take part.

Other 'experts' (such as the builder or a water engineer)

There are many other experts in the community! They may be especially willing to help if they have children in the school. For example, the builder might construct a latrine. The water engineer might arrange for piped water to be laid on to the school (perhaps with help from the community).

All these people may have skills or resources to help the health education programme. Try to use their skills. Bring them into the school. They will improve the school's contact with the community. They will probably learn as much as the pupils learn from them.

Visit the children's homes

The communication between school and community should be a two-way process. Just as you encourage the community to take part in the life of the school, so you can make contact with the children's families. If a child is sick, you can visit the parents. You may be able to explain the cause of the sickness and advise the parents what to do.

You will also have many informal contacts with children's families. With tact, these contacts may provide opportunities to make important points about healthy living. For example, you may be able to explain that diseases have natural causes – and not supernatural ones! Remember what we said about the importance of example at the beginning of this chapter. People will believe your explanations and suggestions if they see that you and your family are healthy people.

The children will take attitudes back to their homes. Thus, when you teach about health, you are teaching the parents of children also. If children develop healthy attitudes, this will affect their parents. Perhaps even more importantly, as we saw in Chapter 9, older children can be encouraged to look after younger children. This is a most valuable channel of communication for good health practices.

Organise a local Health Education Committee

Through cooperative action, you can achieve much more than through individual action. You need the help of other people in the community.

An effective health education committee might consist of the following people:

- the village (or community) Chief or Leader
- the Medical Assistant or Community Health Worker
- religious leaders
- a representative from the parents
- the head-teacher of the school
- a teacher especially interested in health education

In different communities, different people may be interested to sit on the committee. The main aim would be to promote the health of the community, especially the health of the children. If a school management committee already exists, perhaps special meetings could be devoted to health matters in the school and community.

There are many ways in which the committee could work. It might be best to begin with a practical project involving cooperative effort.

Possibilities might include:

- building a special school latrine
- provision of first aid kits
- digging out the drainage ditches around the school

It is best not to be too ambitious at first. Try to get a project going which has a good chance of success.

Children – especially older children – from the school can help in these projects. However, it is important that they do not see themselves as a 'labour gang'. Encourage them to help as willing members of the community. They are more likely to volunteer to help if they understand the **purpose** of the project.

If the committee is effective, it can widen its approach. For example, it could cooperate with the Community Development Officer, the local authority or local Ministry of Health.

It can also press for action. Maybe there is no dispensary. Maybe the dispensary attendant is poorly qualified. The committee could press the local government to take action, and persuade them to provide a dispensary. Or persuade them to send the dispensary attendant for more training. Best of all, persuade them to set up a **child health clinic** (an 'under-fives clinic'). They are for children who are less than five years old – and, of course, for their mothers. Clinics like these have greatly improved the health of young children:

- they are cheap to run
- they aim to teach mothers to care for their children
- if possible, they also look after pregnant mothers (they offer family planning services)
- they are for all children, both healthy and sick . . . not just the sick

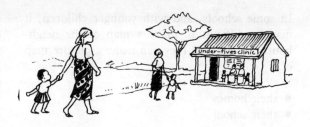

Remember

The best way of improving the health of the community is to improve the health of children. The 'under-fives' clinic is an excellent place to begin.

Map the community

Children could make a health map of the village or community. One is shown here.

Children need to discuss what the map should show. They can decide what are the main health hazards. The map can show what action the community might take to make the village more healthy. Children could identify:

- areas where animals and insects which spread diseases live
- areas where accidents could easily happen to young children
- areas which are dirty and unpleasant
- main landmarks

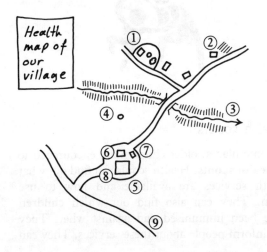

Health map of our village

① my house (prevent accidents)

② market (keep clean)

③ stream (clear snails)

④ well (fence off)

⑤ high grass (cut down)

⑥ school (sweep classrooms)

⑦ kitchen (kill flies)

⑧ school garden (grow vegetables)

⑨ main road (remember safety drill)

In some schools, and with younger children, it may be difficult to make a map of the neighbourhood. Instead they can make a picture map of:

- their homes
- their school
- the way to school

Parents will like to look at these at open days or when they come to the school.

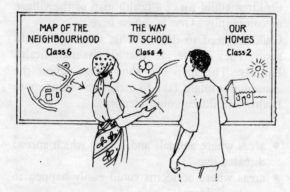

Using the map

Children could look at their map and talk about what they have found. They need time to discuss what can be done and by whom. The children may decide that action should be taken by different groups within the community.

Children, themselves, could tell other children in the school about their work. Children could try to make the school a healthier place. They could clear insect breeding places. They could talk with their parents about how improvements were made in the community in the past. Children could talk with teachers about what the school could do if teachers and pupils worked together.

The community could help through community action. People often have to tell government officials about their neeeds. Role-play and drama can help children to understand how people in

communities make decisions. For example, the children can assume roles as farmers, healthworkers, elders, young teachers, policemen. They could hold council meetings where they discuss village health problems.

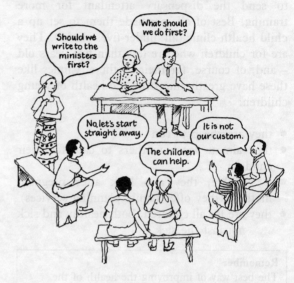

This is a good activity for using the CHILD-to-child idea. Children could discuss how they can help younger children to understand and help.

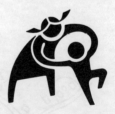

Health scouts

In some places, older children are encouraged to be **health scouts**. Health scouts can find out what health services are available and how to use them. They can also find out which children have been immunised and against what. They can inform people about these services. They can help to care for the health of others, especially younger children. For example:

- The children could make a health services map of the community. On it, they could mark where to go for help. They could work out the travelling time needed to get to each helper.

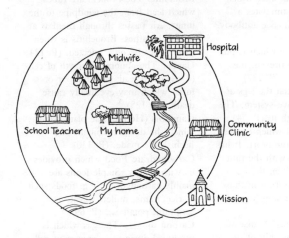

Health Map for our Village
The circles represent each hour's walk from School or Home

- If the health worker is holding a clinic in the village, each scout could be responsible for telling several households.
- Health scouts could become helpers at the health clinic. They might make toys and games for child minders. They might bring young children to the health clinic. They might make health posters and notices.
- They could carry out surveys of local medicines which are used. They could find out what bad accidents occur in the area and tell the health worker.

A school health convention

The school could decide that a special day in the year should be set aside for a **health convention**. All the children's work on health could be put on display. Games and physical education displays could be organised. Parents and community leaders could be invited. The members of the community health committee should be involved in the organisation.

Games and sports would be an important part of the day. However, it is important that the day is not merely a sports day but a day which concentrates on all aspects of health.

Children could perform plays to illustrate important health ideas. If the health committee is interested, adults from the community might also perform short plays. Remember that the plays should be entertaining even if they do contain an important message. People will need time to discuss the plays afterwards.

A partnership for health

Schools and teachers sometimes overestimate their importance in the education of children! For school is not the only place where children learn. Both at home, and in the village or town where they live, children are learning all the time. Teachers can help to encourage a partnership between the school, children's homes, and the wider community. This applies in most aspects of education but especially in health. The school cannot do all the work by itself.

In many place in the world, disease, disability, and death are a distressingly familiar feature of people's lives. Education about health is therefore of direct and immediate relevance. Perhaps health education presents the best opportunity for the school to reach out beyond its doors – to touch and involve the wider community. This demands that teachers should show vision, skill and effort. But it will be worth it if children's lives are enriched and saved.

Glossary

The page references at the end of each entry indicate where the word is mentioned in the text. An asterisk (*) by a word means that it is explained in this glossary.

Abdomen In man, it is the hollow part of the body which is below the chest and above the legs. It contains the stomach, intestines, and many other organs. (P. 60, 75)

Addict A person who is used to taking a drug (e.g. heroin) and cannot do without it is an addict. The person is said to be addicted. (P. 128)

Adolescence The years between about 13 and 19 in a person's life. It is the time between puberty (*) and adulthood. (P. 59)

Alcohol A substance which is present in drinks such as wine, beer, whisky. An alcoholic is a person who overuses alcohol and cannot do without it. (P. 126)

Anaemia A condition where the blood has too few red blood cells. The person looks tired, is pale, and has little energy. (P. 71)

Anaesthetic A substance which prevents the body from feeling pain, heat and cold. It is sometimes injected into the blood. Sometimes it is given as a gas. (P. 129)

Antibiotic A medicine which fights diseases caused by bacteria (*). It has little effect on diseases caused by viruses (*), or fungi (*). (P. 84)

Antibody A substance which is produced by the body in reaction to an antigen (*). The antibody combines chemically with the antigen and makes it harmless. (P. 87)

Antigen A foreign substance which enters the body and stimulates a chemical reaction to it. See antibody (*) above. (P. 87)

Antiseptic A substance which is put on cuts or wounds to prevent the growth of bacteria (*). (P. 137)

Anus The hole between the legs at the end of the digestive system. The faeces (*) pass through it. (P. 74)

Artery A blood vessel which carries blood (*) away from the heart. It has thick walls compared with the thin walls of a vein (*). When the heart beats, you can feel the beat in those arteries just under the skin (e.g. of the wrist). (P. 39)

Athlete's foot A fungus (*) disease which often affects the skin of the feet. It makes the skin itch. (P. 84)

Bacteria These are tiny living things which cannot be seen without a microscope. They cause many infectious diseases. (P. 83) Not all bacteria are 'bad' (some help in the decomposition of dead plants and animals).

Bilharzia A disease which is caused by a worm which gets into the blood. The most common sign is that the person has blood in the urine. (P. 94)

Bladder The bag below the kidneys (*) where urine (*) is stored. (P. 61)

Blood The liquid which carries food, oxygen (*), carbon dioxide (*) and waste products around the body. It contains different cells (red and white cells) which have different functions. Blood passes around the body in blood vessels: arteries (*), veins (*), and capillaries (very small blood vessels). (P. 38)

Bronchitis The bronchi are tubes which lead from the windpipe to the lungs. Air passes through them as a person breathes. Bronchitis is when these tubes become infected. (P. 124)

Cancer The abnormal growth of cells (*). It often leads to a tumour or lump which may eventually cause death. (P. 125)

Cannabis (Hemp) The plant from which the drugs marijuana and hashish are made. (P. 130)

Carbohydrate Food which provides us with energy. Staple foods are mainly carbohydrate (e.g. foods such as rice, yams, millet, wheat, sorghum, potatoes). (P. 69)

Carbon dioxide The gas which is produced during the process of cell respiration. The air which we breathe out contains much more carbon dioxide than the air which we breathe in. (P. 36)

Carbon monoxide A poisonous gas which is found, for example, in cigarette smoke. It affects the ability of the blood to carry oxygen (*). (P. 123)

Carnivore An animal which eats other animals. (P. 33)

Cell Plants and animals are made up of tiny 'building blocks' called cells. They can be seen only through a microscope. Some living things have only one cell but a tree or human being has many millions of cells. (P. 37)

Chickenpox This is a disease which often affects children. It is caused by a virus (*) which produces a rash of red, itchy spots. The rash goes away in a week. (P. 84)

CHILD-to-child A programme which has produced materials, especially in health education, to help older children to look after their younger brothers and sisters. (P. 163)

Cholera An infectious disease which causes vomiting and diarrhoea. It is spread by flies and dirty water. (P. 85)

Cilia These are tiny thread-like structures which are on the surface of certain cells (*) (e.g. the cells lining the trachea (*)). They beat in a regular way, moving the liquid past the cell. (P. 124)

Cocaine A dangerous drug which is used as a stimulant by drug addicts (*). (P. 129)

Condom A contraceptive (*) which a man wears on his penis during sexual intercourse. (P. 64)

Conjunctiva A very thin layer which covers the surface of the eye. (P. 24) Sometimes the conjunctiva become infected, making the eye red and watery. This condition is called conjunctivitis.

Contraceptive A device or a way of preventing pregnancy. (P. 63)

Cornea This is the transparent covering of the surface of the eye. Light passes through it to the back of the eye where it strikes the sensitive retina (*). (P. 24)

Decay This is a chemical process caused by bacteria (*) and fungi (*). It causes dead plants and animals to decompose. It also refers to the rotting of teeth. (P. 32)

Dehydration This is a condition where the body loses more water than it takes in. If the water is not replaced, the person can die. It is especially dangerous for babies. (P. 91)

Dependence A condition where a person has to have a drug for his body to feel normal. (P. 130)

Dermis The innermost layer of cells in the skin. It is much thicker than the epidermis (*). (P. 22, 23)

Diagnose To determine what is wrong with a person by careful observation of their symptoms (*). (P. 101)

Diaphragm A big muscle between the chest and abdomen. It is used in breathing. (P. 38, 39)

Diarrhoea Frequent watery faeces (*). It can cause dehydration (*). (P. 90)

Diet The kinds and amounts of foods which a person should eat (or avoid eating). A balanced diet contains foods of the right kinds in the right amounts. (P. 70)

Digestion The process by which the body breaks food down into simpler substances. This is done by the digestive system. The simpler substances are absorbed into the blood (*) from the intestine (*) which is a part of the digestive system. (P. 74)

Disability Some defect of the body, mind or senses. A disabled person is unable to do those things which other people of their age and sex can do. (P. 48)

Drug A chemical substance which enters the body either through the mouth or through injection into the blood. It affects the physical or mental state of that person. (P. 120)

Embryo The early stage in the development of a baby soon after fertilisation of an egg. (P. 62)

Epidermis The thin outer layer of cells in the skin. (P. 22)

Eustachian Tube The tube which leads from the middle ear to the throat. It allows the air pressure on each side of the ear drum to be the same. (P. 25)

Fallopian Tube A tube which leads from the ovary (*) to the uterus (*). (P. 60, 61)

Faeces Waste food, dead cells and bacteria which pass out from the digestive system. Faeces are sometimes called stools. There are many slang terms for faeces e.g. shit. Defaecation is the process of sending faeces from the body. (P. 75)

Fat A food substance which is rich in energy. It is stored under the skin. (P. 70)

First Aid Emergency care or treatment for a person who is sick or injured. (P. 110)

Fit A fit is when a person has sudden violent convulsions or spasms which he/she cannot control. Sometimes, the person loses consciousness. (P. 49)

Flannel Graph (Flannel Board) A visual aid in which a piece of flannel or rough cloth is stretched over a piece of flat wood or board. Pieces of flannel or rough cloth are then stuck on to the back of drawings enabling the drawings to be stuck with ease to the flannel board. (P. 154)

Fluoride A substance which is necessary for the healthy development of teeth. It can be added to drinking water or toothpaste. (P. 32)

Foetus When an embryo (*) begins to look like a baby, it is called a foetus. This happens about two months after fertilisation. (P. 62)

Fungus A fungus is a kind of plant. It is not green. A mushroom is a fungus. However, there are many fungi (plural of fungus) which are so tiny that they can be seen only with a microscope. Some diseases are caused by fungi, especially diseases of the skin, (see ringworm (*)). (P. 84)

Genital Organs The organs of the reproductive system, (the sex organs). (P. 59)

Germ A very small living thing (bacteria (*), viruses (*), fungi (*)) and one-celled organisms which causes disease. (P. 83)

Gonorrhoea One of the most common of the venereal diseases (*). (P. 96, 97)

Grooming Personal care of the body. (P. 31)

Habit Something which a person does regularly, often without thinking about. (P. 43)

Hallucinogen A drug which causes people to see and feel things in a very strange way. (P. 130)

Health convention We use the term in this book to mean a day when a school concentrates on health and healthy living. Children's work is displayed and parents are invited. (P. 199)

Health scouts Older children can be health scouts. They can find out about health services and health problems. (P. 198)

Health Worker A person who has been given some training in health care and works in rural or poor urban areas. Sometimes they are called medical auxiliaries or barefoot doctors. (P. 195)

Herbivore An animal which eats plants only, not other animals. See also 'carnivore'. (*) (P. 33)

Hookworm A small worm which can pass through the skin and into the blood. Eventually it gets into the intestine and attaches itself to the wall where it lives off the blood of the person. It causes anaemia (*) and general ill health. (P. 89)

Hormones Chemical substances which are produced by various glands of the body. They pass into the blood and act as chemical 'messengers' which have an effect in another part of the body. (P. 59)

Hygiene Practices and actions for healthy living. (P. 88–90)

Iodine A chemical substance which the body needs in very small amounts for its healthy growth and functioning. It is sometimes added to salt. (P. 50, 71)

Immunity The ability of a plant or animal to resist attack by disease organisms. (P. 93)

Kidney There are two kidneys in the body of a human being. They are large organs, shaped like a bean, and lie at the back of the abdomen (*). They filter waste from the blood, forming urine. (P. 94)

Latrine A hole or pit in the ground which is used as a toilet. (P. 185, 186)

Lens In the eye, the lens focuses light on to the retina (*) at the back of the eye. (P. 24)

Lice Small insects which live in the hair or on the body. They cause itching and sometimes skin infections. See also 'nits'. (P. 27)

Liver This is a large organ in the abdomen which helps to clean the blood and has other important functions. (P. 127)

Malaria A kind of fever which is spread by mosquitoes. The mosquitoes inject the germs of malaria when they bite somebody. (P. 92, 93)

Malnutrition This is the condition which occurs when a person does not have enough to eat; or does not have enough of the right kinds of food. (P. 51, 80)

Marijuana (Hashish) This is a drug which is made from the dried leaves and flowers of the hemp (or cannabis) plant. (P. 130)

Measles An infectious disease caused by a virus (*). It often affects children who may die from it. The main signs are fever and skin rash. (P. 96)

Melanin A dark brown or black pigment which is found in the skin. The amount of melanin determines skin colour. (P. 23)

Menopause The time when a woman stops having monthly periods (monthly bleeding). This normally happens between the ages of 40 and 50. (P. 61)

Menstruation The bleeding which takes place approximately every 28 days in women. The bleeding is caused by the breakdown of the wall of the uterus (*) and blood flows out through the vagina (*). (P. 60–63)

Minerals Chemical substances which are required in very small amounts by the body. Examples include iron, iodine (*) and calcium. (P. 69, 70)

Mucous membrane Cells (*) of the body which produce mucus (*). (P. 25)

Mucus A slippery liquid which is produced by the cells which line the mouth, throat, stomach (*), intestines (*), windpipe, and vagina (*). (P. 123, 124)

Mumps A disease which causes painful swelling in the neck. (P. 84)

Navel The belly button. The place where the umbilical cord (*) was attached. (P. 63)

Nicotine A poisonous oily substance which is contained in tobacco leaves. (P. 123, 126)

Night Blindness A condition where a person can see normally during the day but cannot see clearly at night. It is often caused by a lack of vitamin (*) A in the diet. (P. 24)

Nits The eggs of lice. (*) (P. 27)

Nutrient A substance which is used as food by a living organism (*). (P. 69–71)

Nutrition The process in which the body is supplied with food. Nutritious foods are those which the body needs to have energy, grow and stay healthy. (P. 67–81)

Oesophagus or gullet Part of the digestive system. The tube which leads from the mouth to the stomach (*). (P. 75)

Organ A part of the body which has a particular purpose. Lungs, kidneys (*), liver (*) are examples of organs. (P. 39)

Organism A living thing, either plant or animal. (P. 83, 84)

Ossify To become bone. (P. 25)

Ovary Two small organs in the abdomen of a woman which produce eggs. The egg can join with a man's sperm (*) to make a baby. (P. 60–63)

Ovum Egg. (Plural: ova) (P. 60)

Oxygen A gas which is found in air (about 20% of the volume). It is vital for life, and enters the body through the lungs (P. 36–38)

Pancreas An organ of the body in the abdomen (*) which produces a hormone (*) called insulin. (P. 75)

Parasite An organism (*) which lives in or on a person or other animal and causes harm to it. Fleas, lice or worms (such as hookworm (*)) are parasites. (P. 83)

Peer In this book, we have used the word to refer to children of the same age or level. (P. 46)

Penis The male organ between the legs. Urine passes through it to the exterior of the body. It is used in sexual intercourse to put sperm (*) into the woman's vagina (*). (P. 60–64)

Periodontal disease Inflammation of the gums around the teeth. (P. 32)

Pituitary A gland which is part of the brain. It produces several hormones (*) which control many functions of the body. (P. 59)

Placenta A structure in the uterus (*) wall where the foetus (*) joins the mother. The baby receives food and oxygen (*) through the placenta. It normally comes away from the mother about 15 minutes to half an hour after the baby is born. (P. 62, 63)

Plaque Germs on the teeth mix with food and cause a film or coating called plaque. The plaque produces acid which can cause decay of the teeth unless it is removed by brushing. (P. 32, 34)

Pneumonia An acute infection of the lungs. It can be treated with antibiotics (P. 84)

Polio A virus (*) disease which causes paralysis. (P. 51)

Pore A tiny opening in the skin through which sweat passes. (P. 23)

Puberty The stage at which a person becomes sexually mature. (See also adolescence). (P. 59, 60)

Pulse When the heart beats it causes a wave to pass through the blood system of a person. You can feel this wave in any artery (*) near the surface of the body (e.g. the wrist).

If you feel the pulse, you can count how many times a person's heart beats in one minute. (P. 12)

Pupil The round opening or black centre in the middle of the eye. If the light increases, it gets smaller; if the light decreases, it gets larger. (P. 24)

Pus A thick, yellowish white liquid which comes out from a part of the body which is infected. (P. 96)

Rabies A serious disease which is spread by the bite of a dog and some other animals. Once the sickness begins in a person, it is impossible to save his life. (P. 84–86)

Rapid Eye Movement (REM) When a person dreams, his eyes move around under the lids. You can sometimes see these movements if you watch the eyes of a person who is sleeping. (P. 37)

Respiration Breathing. It also means the way cells get energy from food and oxygen. (P. 37–39)

Retina The back inner surface of the eyeball. Light is focussed on to it by the cornea (*) and lens (*). It contains a layer of cells which are sensitive to light. From the retina, nerve impulses are sent to the brain. (P. 24)

Ringworm A fungus infection which affects the skin, causing itching. It often develops in the form of a ring. (P. 27)

River Blindness A disease which is spread by little black flies. The flies inject a worm into a person. The worms can cause small lumps under the skin. If the disease is not treated, the person becomes blind. (P. 24)

Role Play A teaching/learning method where children act out a play. They pretend to be other people and behave and speak like them. (P. 54, 101)

Sanitation Public cleanliness in which the community is involved. Public places are kept clean and free of waste. (P. 184–185)

Scald To burn the skin with hot liquid (e.g. boiling water) or steam. (P. 112)

Scheme of Work A plan which teachers make for the period of a term or school year or over several years in a particular subject. It indicates what subject matter will be covered and in what order. (P. 178)

Sebum The oily substance which is produced by some of the glands of the skin. It helps to keep hair and skin soft and waterproof. (P. 23)

Sedative A drug which calms nerves and reduces stress. (P. 130)

Semen The liquid, produced by men, in which the sperms (*) are contained. (P. 61)

Semi-Circular Canals These are three tubes which are found in the ear. They help the body to balance. (P. 25)

Septic If a wound is septic, it is infected by germs. It often produces pus. (P. 85, 86)

Sleeping Sickness A disease which causes fever and is spread by the tsetse fly. It is common in many parts of Africa. (P. 86)

Spasm A sudden muscle contraction which a person cannot control. Spasms of the jaw and other muscles occur, for example, in tetanus (*). (P. 96)

Spastic Due to brain damage, a spastic person has abnormal muscle contractions. The legs often cross like scissors. (P. 49)

Sperm A man produces sperms in his testes (*). The sperm is tiny and has a 'head' and a 'tail'. With its tail, it can swim up the vagina (*) and uterus (*) of a woman to fertilise an egg (or ovum (*)) which she has produced. Millions of sperms are produced at one time. (P. 61–63)

Staple food The main food which people eat. It provides energy cheaply. Cereals, starchy roots and fruits are the main staple foods of people. (P. 69–71)

Stimulant A drug (*) which makes a person feel lively. It speeds up the activity of the brain. (P. 130)

Stomach The organ in the abdomen (*) in which food is stored when it is eaten. Some digestion (*) of the food takes place in it. Sometimes people use the term stomach to mean the abdomen (*). (P. 75)

Stools Same meaning as faeces (*). (P. 75)

Sweat The salty liquid which is produced by glands in the skin. It helps to keep the body cool. (P. 26)

Symptoms The signs of illness in a sick person. Symptoms provide evidence about a person's illness. (P. 71, 92–97)

Syphilis One of the venereal diseases (*) which affect the sex organs. (P. 96–97)

Tally Chart A convenient way of displaying certain kinds of information. (P. 40)

Tapeworm A parasitic (*) worm which gets into the intestine. You get it if you eat infected beef or pork which is not properly cooked (P. 85)

Tendon A strong cord which attaches a muscle to a bone. (P. 12)

Testes Part of a man's sex organs which lie behind the penis (*). They produce sperms (*) and some hormones (*). (P. 60–62)

Tetanus It is sometimes called lockjaw. It is a disease which is caused by a germ which lives in the faeces (*) of people and animals. The germs often enter through deep and dirty wounds (P. 96)

Toxin Poison. See also 'anti-toxin'. (P. 84)

Trachea The windpipe which leads from the mouth to the lungs. (P. 38)

Trachoma An infection of the conjunctiva (*) of the eye. It slowly gets worse and may result in blindness. (P. 24, 25)

Tuberculosis A serious disease of the lungs. It must be treated as soon as any symptoms appear. It can be prevented by BCG vaccination (*). (P. 93–94)

Typhoid This is a serious disease of the digestive system. It causes high fever after a time. It spreads from faeces to mouth, often in dirty water. (P. 83–88)

Typhus This is an illness which is like typhoid but is not the same. It is spread by lice, ticks and rat fleas. It also causes a fever. (P. 86)

Ulcer A break in the skin or mucous membrane (*). It often lasts a long time. Ulcers may appear on the skin, in the gut or the eye. (P. 125)

Umbilical Cord The cord which connects a baby to its mother in the uterus (*). It goes from the navel on the baby to the placenta (*). (P. 62, 63)

Urine The liquid waste which passes out from the body. (P. 85)

Uterus The womb of a woman. A large muscular organ (*) where the baby develops. (P. 60–64)

Vaccination A medicine which protects a person from specific diseases e.g. polio (*), measles (*), tetanus (*). (Also called immunisation.) (P. 87)

Vagina Birth canal leading from the uterus to the exterior and opening between the legs. (P. 61–65)

Vein A blood vessel which carries blood (*) back to the heart. It has thin walls compared with the thick walls of an artery (*). (P. 39)

Venereal Disease A disease which is spread by sexual contact. (See gonorrhoea and syphilis.) (P. 96, 97)

Virus A very small germ which can cause some very important diseases. Viruses are smaller than bacteria (*). (P. 84–87)

Vitamin Foods which are required in very small quantities for the healthy working of the body. (P. 70)

Whooping Cough A disease of children which can be prevented easily by vaccination (*). The main symptom is a very characteristic cough. (P. 51)

Yellow Fever An infectious tropical disease which causes the skin to turn yellow. (P. 86)

Index

Page references with an asterisk mean that this is the main topic on that page.